ANNE HOOPER'S
ULTIMATE
SEX
GUIDE

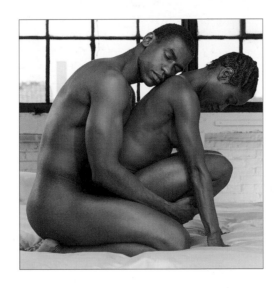

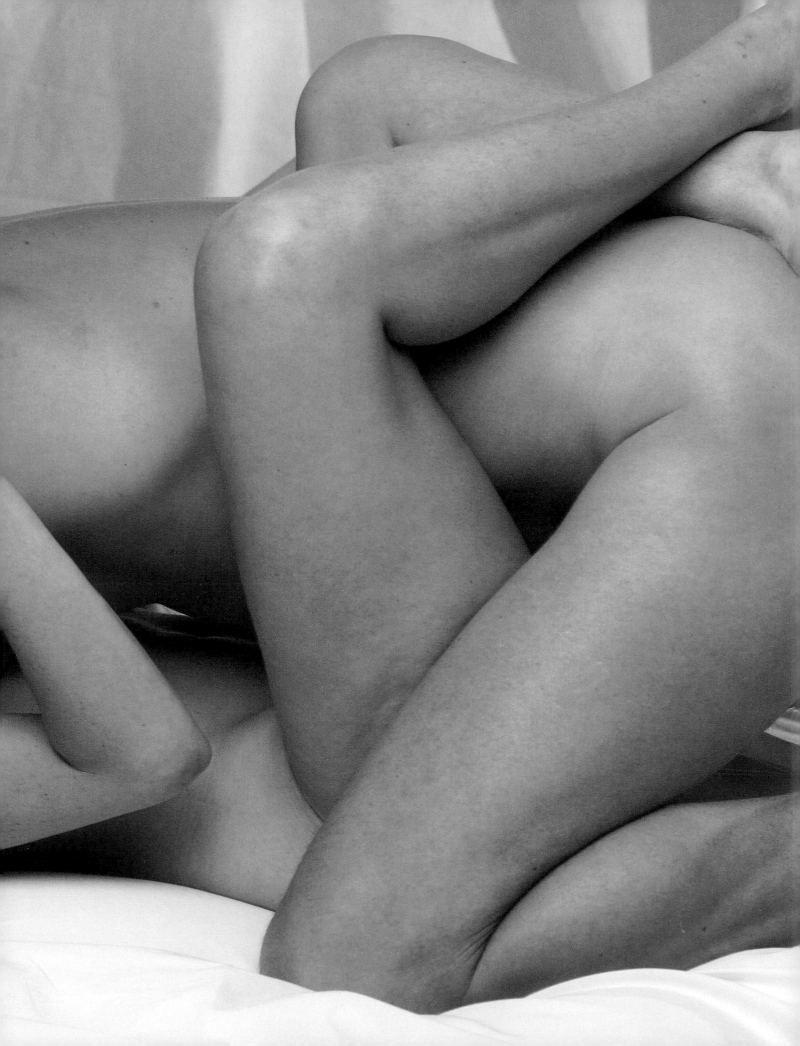

ANNE HOOPER'S

ULTIMATE

SEX GUIDE

*A therapist's guide to the
programs and techniques that will
enhance your relationship and
transform your life*

A DORLING KINDERSLEY BOOK

Dorling 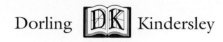 Kindersley

LONDON, NEW YORK, SYDNEY, DELHI,
PARIS, MUNICH, and JOHANNESBURG

Original edition
Created and produced by
CARROLL & BROWN LIMITED

Revised edition
Senior Managing Art Editor Lynne Brown
Senior Managing Editor Corinne Roberts
Senior Art Editor Karen Ward
Senior Editor Julia North
US Editor Margaret Parrish
Production Bethan Blase

First published in Great Britain in 1992
First American edition, 2001

00 01 02 03 04 05 10 9 8 7 6 5 4 3 2 1

Published in the United States by
Dorling Kindersley Publishing, Inc.
95 Madison Avenue, New York, New York 10016

DK publishing offers special discounts for bulk purchases for sales
promotions or premiums. Specific, large-quantity needs can be met
with special editions, including personalized covers, excerpts of existing
guides, and corporate imprints. For more information, contact Special
Markets Department, DK Publishing, Inc., 95 Madison Avenue,
New York, NY 10016 Fax: 800-600-9098

A CIP catalog record for this book is
available from the Library of Congress.

ISBN 0 7894 7265 1

Reproduced by Colourscan, Singapore
Printed in Italy by L.E.G.O.

See our complete catalog at
www.dk.com

FOREWORD

During my years as a sex therapist and as the director of a clinic for sexual problems, I have met with a great variety of people needing to improve and expand their sex lives. The most sensible, intelligent, and successful individuals have attended my practice. Sex problems are not the prerogative of the less able. And sexual curiosity appears to be universal. Everybody wants to know if they can make sex even better than it already is.

Among my clients have been members of government, high-ranking police officers, doctors, psychiatrists, opera singers, musicians, and best-selling novelists. There have also been nurses, teachers, a gourmet chef, dentists, accountants, lawyers, factory workers, the unemployed, garbage collectors, men and women with incurable illnesses, and housewives and househusbands.

I have learned a great deal from my clients during this time – not least of which is that sex is fun. It is also restorative, reassuring, and provides the underpinning for a loving partnership. It is patently *not* unusual to want to learn more about personal sexuality.

Yet, however hard a therapist works and however many clients she manages to see, there is a limit to the number she can reach. In addition, some men and women have a powerful desire to retain their privacy. This means that there are a great many people still longing to know more about their sensual selves, and it is for them that I have written this book.

Good sex consists of feeling alive and well in the brain and awake and on fire in the body. It uses technical skills as well as personal preferences. It is an art, not in the sense of being a dead and artificial art form, but in becoming a unique and creative experience for the two people taking part. Through this book I hope to use my clinical learning to assist such creative experiences. By feeding new thoughts (and occasionally some very old thoughts) to you, I hope you develop a vital, powerful love life. May it provide you with vivid experiences and memories.

Anne Hooper

CONTENTS

INTRODUCTION

Sex has often been referred to as the poor person's pastime — a reference to the fact you don't need to buy anything in order to do it or to enjoy it. We carry within ourselves all the ingredients for ecstasy, and even if we don't have a partner, it is still possible for us to enjoy personally created scenarios of sexual pleasure. But if sex is such a natural resource, why should we bother with books such as this one? Why don't we all glide along in a continual stream of orgasmic rapture doing, quite simply, what comes naturally?

SEX IS AN ACQUIRED SKILL

We often don't make the most of our sexual capacities because our grasp of them is uncertain. Most of us learn about sex from family and friends and the courting examples of our contemporaries. On a wider level, we learn about sex through the media. And, in our bedrooms, we attempt to put into practice the ideas assimilated. Ideally, this happens spontaneously, reenacting playful antics.

Life, however, is not ideal. We may not, in our inhibited Western world, get enough information about sex or enough of the right information. Not everyone has enough power of imagination to use sexual knowledge. Nor will instinct alone guide a person to good sex. Virtually all who reach the heights of bliss do so by accident.

And even if we find we are capable of orgasm, it doesn't automatically entitle us to certified bliss. How often have you felt curiously flat after orgasm? As if there should somehow be more to it? There are never, of course, any guarantees we can reach sexual nirvana, but there are methods that get us close. So one purpose of this book is to provide you with a good start and to increase your satisfaction using, in human terms, all natural ingredients.

TOUCH AND SEXUALITY
Touch is the doorway to stimulation. Through touch we explore our own inner sensation and intimacy with others. As we mature we develop and refine that touch, and sensuality widens into sexuality. This growth is encouraged by curiosity — interest in novelty.

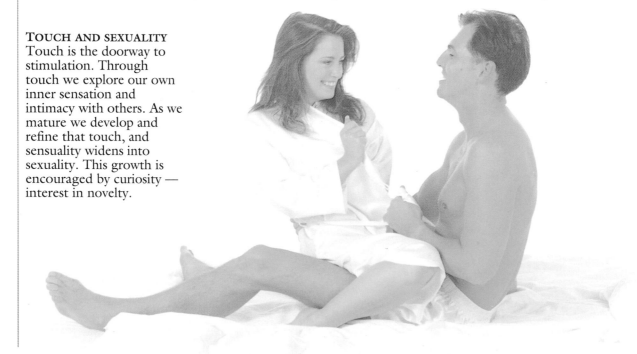

PROBLEMS WITH SEX CAN BE OVERCOME

Being unable to reach one's sexual potential can have long-lasting effects, not only on personal well-being and health but, almost inevitably, on relationships that are the most vital to us. Today, when people seek quality in all aspects of their lives, sexual fulfillment is an area that cannot be overlooked.

Sexual difficulties beset all of us from time to time and, if ignored, can ruin what would otherwise be a major source of satisfaction. Sexual problems are not usually of a great magnitude; most men are not prevented by impotence from engaging in sex, and most women can overcome pain on intercourse. But often an enormous gap exists between what we imagine our sex lives can be and what we manage to achieve.

Sexual difficulties are not new — they've existed as long as people have been engaging in sexual activities — nor are they particularly unique. On the contrary, they are long-standing, clearly identifiable, and extremely prevalent. They are also "curable." Over the years, sexual therapists like me have perfected techniques to tackle the difficulties that clients relate to us day after day. This book contains the programs and practices that can do the greatest possible good. Now readers who can't afford the cost of therapy, or who feel reticent about discussing sexual matters, can, in the privacy of their own homes, discover the ways and means of achieving sexual experiences that live up to their expectations.

A NATURAL APPROACH TO SEX

While I cannot guarantee that on perusal of this book you will automatically experience Grade A ecstasy, I can guarantee that by trying some of the sex programs you will enjoy gorgeous sensuality. Who knows? These items of sex information, factored into your sex play, may trigger a very special erotic experience — one that truly feels like rapture. And it is all done by knowing how to stimulate the natural chemicals of the brain and body.

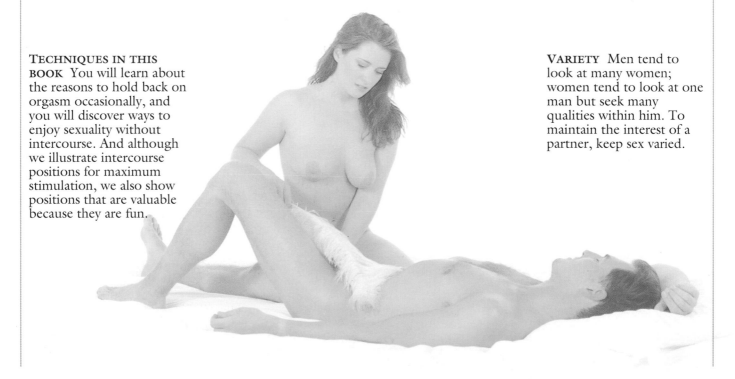

TECHNIQUES IN THIS BOOK You will learn about the reasons to hold back on orgasm occasionally, and you will discover ways to enjoy sexuality without intercourse. And although we illustrate intercourse positions for maximum stimulation, we also show positions that are valuable because they are fun.

VARIETY Men tend to look at many women; women tend to look at one man but seek many qualities within him. To maintain the interest of a partner, keep sex varied.

Few people realize that their bodies are a natural pharmacopeia. During sex we manufacture chemicals that make us feel wonderful. We produce an amazing substance that floods the tissues, allowing us to experience touch with dreamlike sensuality, and we also create, as a by-product of sexual climax, a substance that sends us to sleep, a pleasant, natural relaxant. And parts of the sexual response cycle utilize adrenaline surges, resulting in powerful bursts of energy. These allow us to take great satisfaction from sustained movement of the body, the naturally aerobic spin-off of the sex act.

In addition, our brains are able to send us on journeys into landscape and emotion without help from anything that acts on our bodies from the inside. We can gain other-worldly experience through guided fantasy or fantasy experiments that bring endless variation to sex and sharpen sexual sensation with concentrated intensity.

Children learn about themselves and how to become fully functional human beings through the medium of play, and adults find out about sex in similar fashion. Play isn't just the froth of life; it has purpose. It is a practical way of gaining knowledge and experience, not only of how things work but of how we work. Play is the building block of human experience. Playing, having fun, experimenting, literally fooling around, are all methods of learning about sensuality.

The programs and techniques shown in this book are based on play and on utilizing the natural resources of our sexuality. They have helped hundreds of people turn their insufficiently rewarding or boring sexual relationships into opportunities for uncovering new and exciting feelings in themselves and their partners. And the only necessary ingredients are imagination, erotic touch, and knowledge about our sexual selves.

THE ENDLESS VARIETY OF SEX

Often our sex lives stagnate because the sex act becomes boringly repetitive. The reason for this, ironically, is that when we hit on a good position (or a good combination of fingers and penis) we go back to it increasingly often. After all, we know it works. Yet life often remains interesting because of its uncertainties. Where Sigmund Freud reckoned that sexuality is our motivating life force and Alfred Adler said that a drive for integration is the explanation, I rate the need for survival a more realistic possibility. The drive to survive takes in both sexual urges and social fit, but depends most of all on what I have termed the anti-boredom factor — a drive toward stimulation.

Experimenting with different sex positions, or just looking at pictures of them in a book such as this, offers encouragement to those novelty-seeking brain cells. Indeed, it is by forgetting about the possibilities for sexual permutation that many relationships decline sexually. It's not good enough to explain that by knowing someone so intimately you automatically learn everything about them, and therefore there is nothing new to discover. There is always something new, but you must use your brain to find it. I hope this book is an aid to such sensual creation.

Even if only one basic sex position is favored, it can still be varied by the thoughts or dialogue you choose at the time. Physically, there are alterations to your posture or balance that may not seem especially different but, nevertheless, lead to other thoughts and feelings.

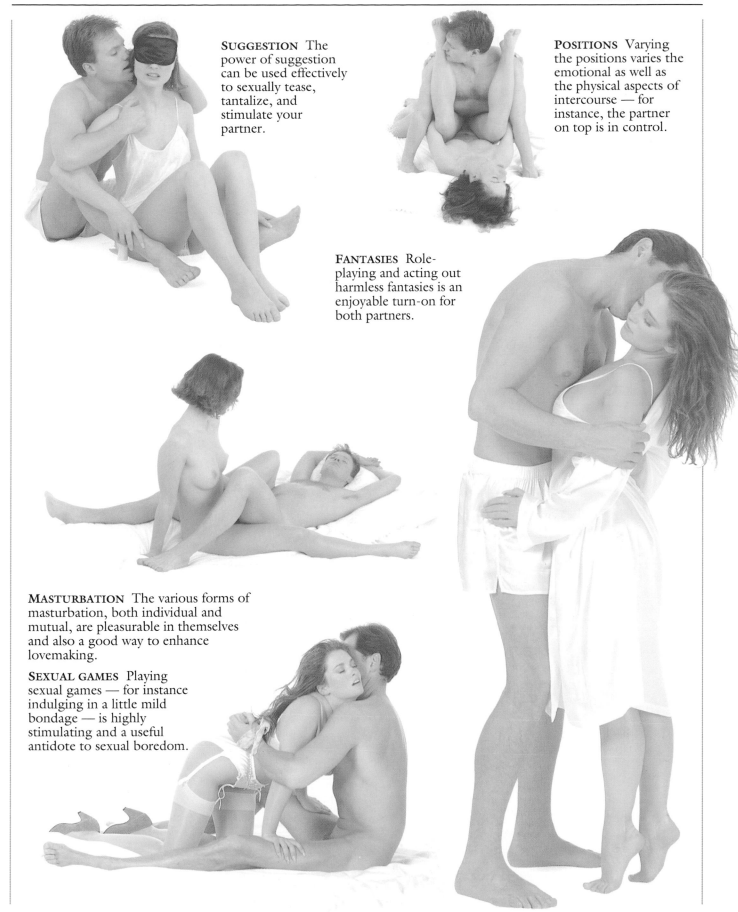

SUGGESTION The power of suggestion can be used effectively to sexually tease, tantalize, and stimulate your partner.

POSITIONS Varying the positions varies the emotional as well as the physical aspects of intercourse — for instance, the partner on top is in control.

FANTASIES Role-playing and acting out harmless fantasies is an enjoyable turn-on for both partners.

MASTURBATION The various forms of masturbation, both individual and mutual, are pleasurable in themselves and also a good way to enhance lovemaking.

SEXUAL GAMES Playing sexual games — for instance indulging in a little mild bondage — is highly stimulating and a useful antidote to sexual boredom.

THE ACT OF SEX

Becoming adept in the arts of sexual loving requires a clear understanding of the way sex works. Many of the difficulties partners face in their sexual activities can be caused by a lack of information about what happens during sex and, even more, how each partner responds and to what stimuli. Men and women share similarities of sexual response, but they see sex and attraction differently, and their needs don't always correspond. If taken as a process, the sex act has four distinct phases — arousal, penetration, climax, and resolution. Each phase may exist separately from the others, although at the best of times, the phases flow in a continuum. Unless we understand our readiness for and responses to each phase, our ability to have good sex — and sometimes any sex at all — will be seriously undermined.

AROUSAL

In order to want to have sex, a feeling of desire has to be experienced. Arousal appears to originate in the brain, though the phenomenon is still not completely understood, and hormones play an important part. When a man first experiences arousal his penis hardens and becomes erect; a woman's initial response is a moistening of her vagina. As desire increases with the exchange of a variety of caresses and the stimulation of erogenous areas, various other changes occur to both internal and external sexual organs. As desire reaches a peak, both partners long for penetration.

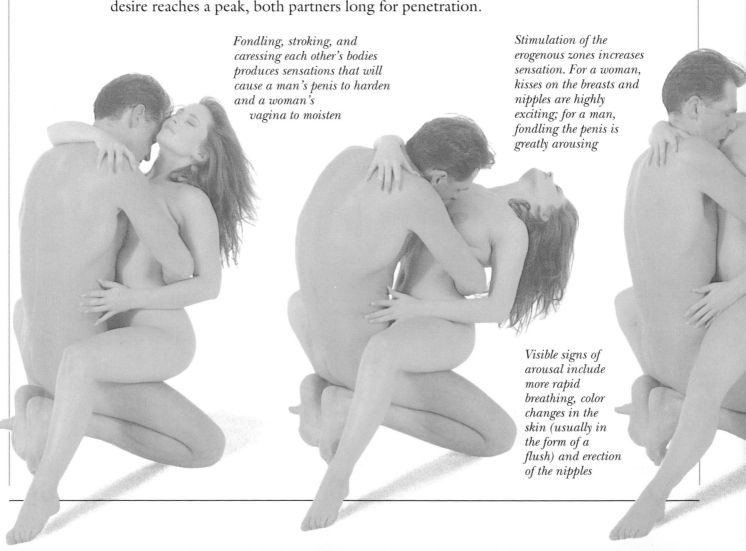

Fondling, stroking, and caressing each other's bodies produces sensations that will cause a man's penis to harden and a woman's vagina to moisten

Stimulation of the erogenous zones increases sensation. For a woman, kisses on the breasts and nipples are highly exciting; for a man, fondling the penis is greatly arousing

Visible signs of arousal include more rapid breathing, color changes in the skin (usually in the form of a flush) and erection of the nipples

PENETRATION

Foreplay should have prepared the vagina and penis sufficiently for penetration; the vagina must be lubricated by its secretions in order to receive a fully erect penis without discomfort. The vagina envelops the penis, and thrusting movements of the penis in this confined space produce sensations throughout both partners' bodies that lead to further internal and external changes, most particularly swelling of the genitals and muscular tensions. These, in turn, lead to feelings of such sexual excitement that, particularly for the man, a climax generally results.

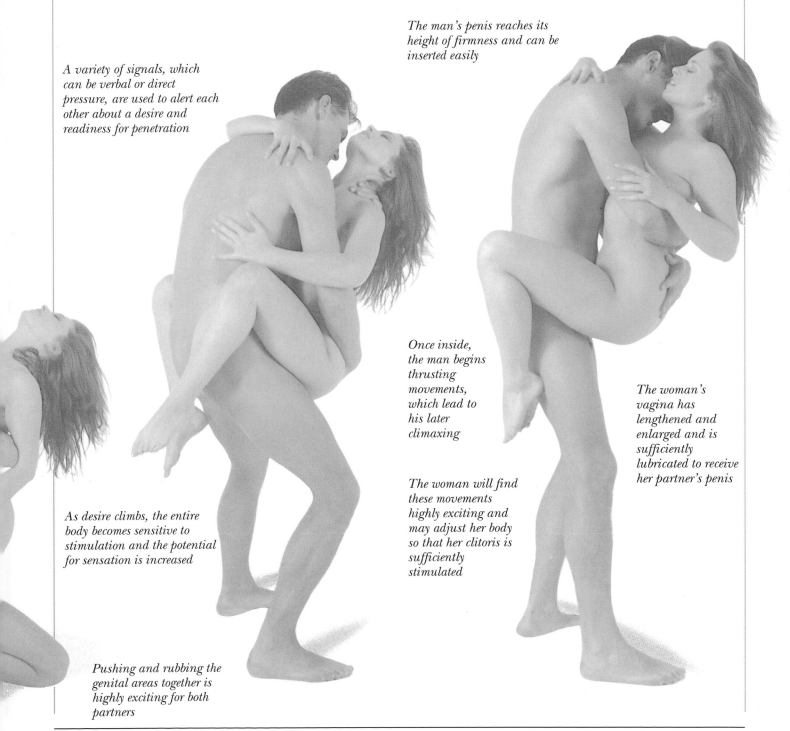

The man's penis reaches its height of firmness and can be inserted easily

A variety of signals, which can be verbal or direct pressure, are used to alert each other about a desire and readiness for penetration

Once inside, the man begins thrusting movements, which lead to his later climaxing

The woman's vagina has lengthened and enlarged and is sufficiently lubricated to receive her partner's penis

As desire climbs, the entire body becomes sensitive to stimulation and the potential for sensation is increased

The woman will find these movements highly exciting and may adjust her body so that her clitoris is sufficiently stimulated

Pushing and rubbing the genital areas together is highly exciting for both partners

ORGASM

When sensations become overwhelmingly intense, both partners experience a peak of pleasure which, with men, is almost inevitably accompanied by the ejaculation of seminal fluid. A man's orgasm depends almost entirely on having his penis stimulated manually, orally, or by the vaginal walls. A woman's orgasm, whether or not she achieves one, and how long it takes to do so, depends very much on the amount of stimulation her clitoris receives. This is a woman's primary organ of sensation. Again, stimulation can be manual or oral, direct or indirect, but direct clitoral stimulation brings the greatest and quickest response.

Rapid thrusts of the penis lead to regularly recurring contractions of the man's urethra and this, in turn, produces the highly pleasurable sensations associated with, though not dependent on, ejaculation. As the seminal fluid is spurted out through the engorged penis via the prostate and urethra, most men experience a powerful physical reaction. A man's orgasm is almost always preceded by a feeling of ejaculatory inevitability, and once he ejaculates, his orgasm cannot be delayed until emission has been completed.

As orgasm approaches, the man's pushing becomes more rhythmic and urgent, and his heart rate and breathing become more rapid

A woman's pleasure proceeds in steplike fashion with that of her partner, her responses keeping time with his thrusting

During the most intense moments of lovemaking, the man's sensations are concentrated on being able to thrust deep inside his partner

Just before the emission of the seminal fluid, the man passes the point of no return, when he can no longer delay climax

The woman's muscles contract and grip the man, and there is an increased blood supply to the vagina

At the moment of climax, intense sensual feelings flood the vaginal area and spread throughout the woman's body

Like her partner, a woman also experiences orgasmic contractions, similar in number and duration, and often at the same intervals. The sensation of orgasm may differ, however, from woman to woman, some experiencing a single peak of pleasure, others having more widespread sensations that can be rekindled, producing more than one orgasm.

RESOLUTION

Once climax occurs, sexual tension falls away. A man experiences an almost immediate drop in sensation; his penis becomes flaccid, and it will be some time before he can become erect again. This is known as the refractory period. After climax, a man normally feels relaxed and sleepy and often, depending on the circumstances, falls into a deep slumber.

For a woman, the return to normality is much slower. She experiences a slow and gradual decline in the swelling of her breasts and labia, and she remains in a responsive state for much longer, even welcoming further loving attentions from her partner.

It should be apparent, therefore, that although men and women are similar in their responses to sex, significant differences exist, particularly as regards arousal and the experience of orgasm. Often, too, we are in such a hurry for orgasm that we lose out on arousal. Yet it is the magic of this stage, that time when we are stimulated to a peak of sexual excitement, that helps the brain leap into a heightened consciousness. It is important that partners be aware of these differences and that they use the techniques shown in this book to give each other the best chance of a totally satisfying sexual life.

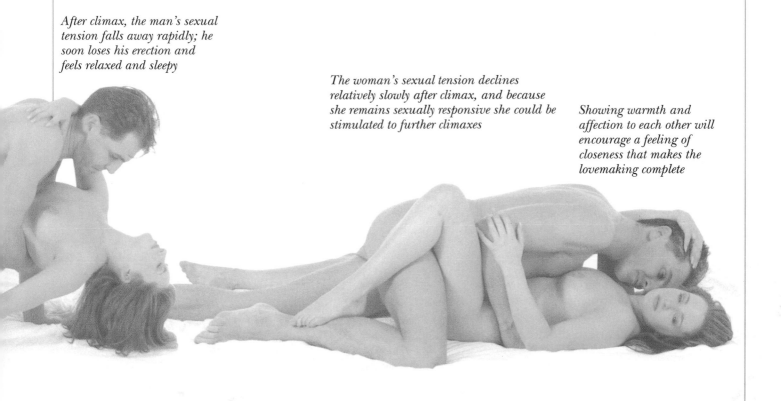

After climax, the man's sexual tension falls away rapidly; he soon loses his erection and feels relaxed and sleepy

The woman's sexual tension declines relatively slowly after climax, and because she remains sexually responsive she could be stimulated to further climaxes

Showing warmth and affection to each other will encourage a feeling of closeness that makes the lovemaking complete

HOW THE BOOK WORKS

Many people express the opinion that sexuality only has value if it is worked out in private, solely between the two people involved. This, however, is faulty reasoning. Sex therapy, far from creating an artificial edge to the rapport between people, assists men and women in experiencing new thoughts and emotions as well as good physical sensations. Here, I offer assistance to all the thousands of people who choose not to meet a therapist face to face but who nevertheless look forward to resolving their sex problems. If you can make full use of the ideas, training methods, and therapeutic discussion I have gathered and developed over the years, I sincerely hope you will be able to enhance your loving relationship in every way.

The Ultimate Sex Book has been compiled to provide you with all the information you need to enhance or improve any sexual relationship. All the areas that are problematical for couples are covered in a similar, easy-to-follow way. Each single question such as "How can I make lovemaking more intimate?" is explored from several angles. For example, in that specific case history, the innermost anxieties and desires that we all may have are communicated safely through the circumstances of one couple in particular. In my assessment of the couple's problem, I explain how emotional intimacy can be fostered, and in the accompanying program I set out a series of simple exercises that encourage physical intimacy. Finally, the program is supplemented by the illustrated exercise that follows it; this provides detailed pictorial instruction of an enjoyable form of touch therapy that will allow you to develop intimate sensual knowledge of each other.

THE CASE HISTORIES

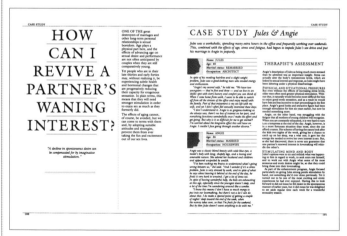

Throughout the pages of this book are case histories taken from my files, each specifically illustrating the sexual yearning and ambition every individual possesses but few care to admit to. The lovers on these pages are not struggling with premature ejaculation or inability to experience orgasm, but they do ask simple questions that sometimes lead to profound answers. "How can I achieve a deeper orgasm?" provokes, for example, a complicated answer because it concerns stimulating the mind.

The people whose problems I have concentrated on here encompass single men and women as well as those in short-term, long-term, and/or conjugal relationships. The age range is wide, too. This only reinforces the truth that disappointment with sexual experiences affects everyone at some time.

These seemingly personal cases do in fact have implications for us all. I have tried in my assessments to generalize from particular circumstances so that anyone reading the case histories would be able to pick up insights into aspects of their own behavior, and so perhaps be furnished with ways of adjusting that behavior for the better.

THE PROGRAMS

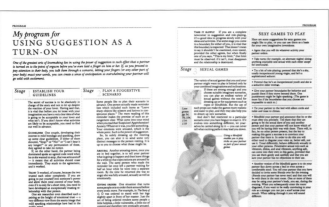

Succeeding each case history are the therapy pages, where a sequence of "stages" to deal with the problem are outlined. The different stages include techniques involving specific mood training, factual information, and touch maneuvers.

In the early pages I deal with issues such as self-esteem and assertion, outlining simple confidence-building exercises for men and women. The connection between confidence and sexuality may not be an obvious one, but it does exist. Having the courage to ask for what you want in lovemaking and the language in which to do it tactfully may, for some couples, be the deciding factor in the rise or fall of a relationship.

The latter pages help expand imagination by helping partners to explore each other's fantasies and by showing how to focus single-mindedly on expanding sensation and consciousness. In this way, the brink of orgasm and orgasm itself can become spiritual ecstasy. No one, of course, can experience ecstasy to order. But by laying the foundations, you have a greater chance of getting there than by leaving it to chance.

Each program is directed toward a particular aspect of sexuality; some deal with mental attitudes, others with physical improvements through mastering specific, proven techniques. Programs may be for individuals or involve a partner. Each program normally involves several stages. This is part of the philosophy and practice of sexual therapy: that improvements happen over time and as the result of building on previous experiences.

ILLUSTRATED EXERCISES

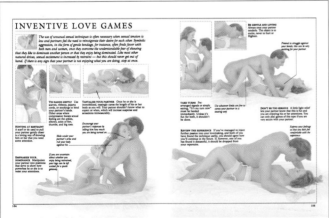

Each program is made up of one or more exercises, which are illustrated methods of lovemaking. I have made certain that the techniques are presented in such a way so as to be accessible and helpful to all. The captions and annotation will guide you through the various stages and draw your attention to the finer points of the techniques so that what is shown can be achieved.

These illustrated exercises are widely applicable to a variety of situations and, while you will get the most value from the book if you read it through fully, you can, should you prefer, work from it using only the exercises.

I have personally seen hundreds of couples rekindle feelings of love while technically carrying out their sex therapy "homework" for me. The facts are that some people need help and instruction even for sex and that therapists, like me, using our expertise and sensitivity, try to give it.

MAKING THE BOOK WORK FOR YOU

In *The Ultimate Sex Book* I have drawn on my fifteen years of practice as a sex therapist. In creating it I have borne the following three issues clearly in mind, and it is extremely important that you do the same.

• It is important to put aside the notions of what you think is allowed between two people in bed, and to embrace the thought that many alternative sex practices may be enjoyed, always providing, of course, you do not cause harm to anyone. *It is possible to change your beliefs.*

• Because of AIDS, it makes a great deal of sense to improve an existing relationship rather than treating it lightly. Bringing warmth, sensuality, and sexual and emotional gratification to lovemaking offers optimum incentive to stay with the same person.

• Focusing simultaneously on sexual *and* emotional issues is a pathway to feeling alive in either an existing or a new relationship. If you can be truly intimate with each other, it's hard to find yourself on "automatic pilot" in bed, and it is far less likely that you will become bored.

YOUR GUIDE TO BETTER SEX

On the simplest level, here you will find an enormous range of mental and physical practices that will expand your repertoire of lovemaking. And that, in itself, is nothing to sneeze at.

Perhaps one or more of the questions posed by the case histories may have a particular resonance for you, and may provide a very specific answer. Do not be put off, however, if the individual circumstances do not exactly mirror yours, or if the recommended programs in their entirety may not, or cannot, be followed as outlined. They are there to illustrate the range of the possible, and even in isolation can help to liberate feelings and transform sexual behavior.

Make sure, however, you involve your partner fully in all these endeavors. In this work, a relationship is any encounter between two people, be it the first one, a casual one, or a long-term series of encounters. In case you argue against the feasibility of a first-time meeting or casual acquaintance amounting to a relationship, there are undoubtedly people who enjoy great emotional heights of sexuality in precisely these situations.

This is not to argue for the constant pursuit of new partners. While it is true that novelty is a powerful aphrodisiac, so too is that marvelous inspiration between man and woman where you know each other's eroticism so intently you are aroused by merely looking at each other. And AIDS is now such a risk it can no longer be wise to opt for novelty when it may end up killing you.

Since this is a work about sex, many of the solutions and techniques proposed in the case studies and on the sex program pages are physical ones. But they are physical solutions that give rise to feelings. The feelings then feed back into lovemaking so that the sex act is enhanced and the relationship itself strengthened.

THE CASE HISTORIES, PROGRAMS, AND EXERCISES

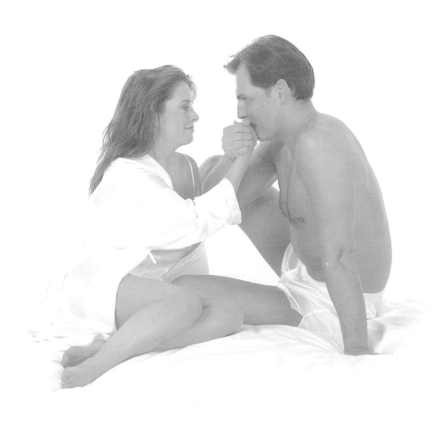

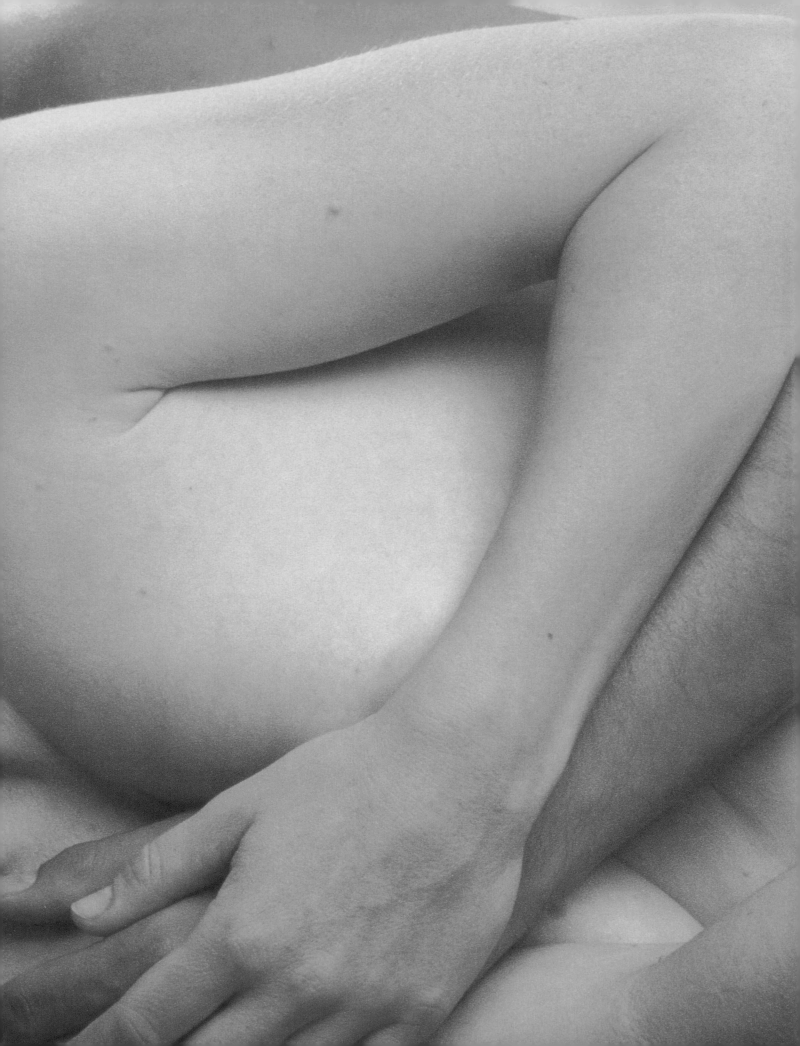

CHAPTER 1

HOW CAN I SHOW MY INTEREST IN SEX?

"For some people, meeting potential partners is easy, but developing the relationship is a problem. For others, the difficulty lies in meeting suitable partners in the first place."

A SEX THERAPIST deals with all aspects of relationships, even the initiation of them. Some people find their main problem with sex is a lack of it, caused by an inability to attract a partner or, having attracted one, being unable to keep them interested.

Men and women, as you can see from my case notes opposite, often have quite different hang-ups about their appearance and behavior that get in the way of successfully communicating their interests and desires. For example, many men erroneously believe that women are attracted by large penis size and a muscular body, while in fact, most women are repelled by these attributes but appreciate small but sexy buttocks, a flat stomach, long legs, and someone taller or of a similar size and build. And while men rate a woman's looks as the most important aspect of her attractiveness, different types of men are attracted to different types of figure and coloring.

Of course, physical attraction alone is not enough to sustain a close long-term relationship — there must also be an emotional and intellectual dimension. So someone who wants to find a new partner for a lasting relationship should pay attention not only to their physical appearance, but also to the way in which they behave and the impression of themselves that they convey to other people.

CASE STUDY *Steve & Caroline*

Finding a suitable partner and starting an intimate relationship is difficult for many people. For some, such as Steve, meeting potential partners is easy, but developing the relationship is a problem. For others, such as Caroline, the difficulty lies in meeting suitable partners in the first place.

Name:	STEVE
Age:	31
Marital status:	SEPARATED
Occupation:	ACCOUNTANT

Steve had recently separated from his wife after an eight-year marriage. Although he already possessed many of the physical characteristics that initially appeal to women – he was tall, well-built, and in good physical shape – he also projected an air of confident indifference that, in fact, obscured his shyness and relative sexual inexperience. He told me, "I find myself wanting to make love to attractive women but without too much success. Women usually appear to be interested in me when we first meet, but only occasionally do we manage to end up in bed together. Inevitably, however, it seems that somehow I do something to frighten them off very quickly.

"What do I have to do to not only get women into bed with me but to help my partners relax, so that we can have really great sex?"

Name:	CAROLINE
Age:	23
Marital status:	SINGLE
Occupation:	EDITOR

Caroline's one long relationship, which lasted about three years, had ended about a year before she came to see me. After it ended she had dated several men, none of whom interested her especially. She was a slim, quiet woman, with glasses, who was efficient and intelligent. She dressed in well-cut but discreet clothes and talked easily when addressed but did not volunteer information. She said, "I am impatient with the men who ask me out; most of them don't seem to have a brain. I rarely come across someone who is my intellectual equal. There is one man at the office whom I find attractive; unfortunately he hardly knows I'm alive.

"I know my upbringing holds me back from flirting, but I think that underneath I'm really a very sexy person. I have terrible hang-ups about my breasts because they're not very big, but I've got nice long legs and I feel I have a lot to offer the right man."

THERAPIST'S ASSESSMENT

What both Steve and Caroline needed to do was to project themselves in a sexier manner.

ATTRACTIVENESS
We all give off distinct impressions of ourselves, usually quite unconsciously, by the way we use body language and by our lifestyles and how we present ourselves. A zest for life, creativity, sexual interest, curiosity, and enjoyment are all extremely attractive. Steve's zest for life certainly wasn't apparent in initial conversations, and he only showed it when talking about his special interest in life — gymnastics.

Contrary to what Steve had originally believed, women are not initially attracted by outstanding looks and physique or even smooth talk. The surest way to become attractive to women is to treat them as alluring human beings rather than as convenient sex objects: no woman is the least bit interested in being just another notch on someone's bedpost.

Caroline was right to target her physical appearance, because this is what men are most attracted to. They respond far more to visual signals than women do, so the value of dressing seductively cannot be overestimated.

LOOKING FOR PARTNERS
My immediate recommendation, therefore, was for Steve to use his sports enthusiasms for breaking the social ice. His shyness would automatically be lifted, and gymnastics would allow his body language to reflect his more confident feelings about this aspect of his life.

I advised Caroline that she was going to need a partner who could deal with her intelligence instead of being intimidated by it, and that she must visit places where she was likely to come into contact with such individuals, perhaps putting herself in the path of men several years older than herself. She should display her figure more too, in particular her long, shapely legs, by wearing tighter-fitting clothes and shorter skirts.

Nor did she have to resort to flirting. Being able to gaze at someone and be genuinely interested in their personal story makes an excellent substitute, and providing information that forms a common ground and facilitates interest is a sensible move to make. Matching a potential partner's story with a similar one would show him that Caroline had emotions and a life experience similar to his, and would let him see that she was being open with him.

My program for PROJECTING A SEXY IMAGE

Part of what is conventionally thought of as being "respectable" behavior lies in sober dress: if you want to seem discreet and unobtrusive, you dress quietly. The trouble with this is that, over the years, you can get used to the idea of yourself as quietly unattractive. However, the opposite is also true — gradually altering your appearance and your body language so that you experience yourself as an erotic individual can be a valuable method of overcoming inhibition. Once you have attracted someone with your appearance, you can use suggestive body language to reinforce the beginnings of sexual attraction, and then use touch to communicate your interest to your prospective partner.

Stage 1 PAY ATTENTION TO YOUR APPEARANCE

Becoming truly sensual is a result of internal changes that alter your attitude to sensuality, but these changes are easier to accommodate and can be speeded up if you tackle your outer sexuality first. Actually putting on a sexier expression as you gaze into a mirror allows you to feel sexier; altering your appearance slowly allows you time to get used to the change. Once you start noticing this change, other people will notice it too. The key to changing outward appearance is to take it gradually. Make one change every couple of weeks or so, and don't be afraid to experiment. And don't give up.

Stage 2 USE BODY LANGUAGE THAT IS SUGGESTIVE

Watch yourself the next time you meet someone new. The odds are that your arms will be folded, or your hands clasped in front of you. If seated, you may have swiveled sideways to avoid directly facing your acquaintance. If you are anxious, one leg may be draped over the other, maybe even wrapped around it. Or you may be huddled back in a corner looking as though you are trying to get as far away from people as possible.

BARRIER SIGNALS All these postures are barrier signals indicating that you feel tense or nervous or even under attack. To the person you are with, they show that you don't welcome them and you don't want them to come near. And even though we don't usually analyze the body language of the person opposite, and may in fact be unaware of it on a conscious level, our subconscious still takes in the messages being given and makes us respond accordingly.

If you want to make someone feel welcome, you need to be open to them. Avoid barrier signals. If you are standing, put your arms at your sides. Keeping your shoulders back and leaning forward slightly can indicate that someone has all your attention but that you

WARMTH MOVES

- Look longer than normal into a partner's eyes.

- Move toward the other person somewhat more than you would normally.

- Smile more than usual, looking in turn at various parts of the body.

- Nod your head in vigorous agreement.

- Sit using open body signals.

- When talking, use hand gestures that manage to take in the partner or that indicate an appreciation of him or her.

- Take fast glances at the other person and while doing so, moisten your lips with your tongue, widening your eyes a little.

- Make small touching movements. For example, when standing together, stand behind your partner cuddling lightly against his or her body, with both arms around the waist; put an arm around your partner; caress and massage your partner's back.

want them to notice you. If you know someone slightly, don't be afraid of hugging them or even casually resting an arm across their shoulders. These are displays of warmth.

If you are seated, resting your arms on the arms of the chair or extending your arms along the back of a sofa are indications that you are open to the person opposite. If you want them to feel in charge of the situation, ensure that they sit in a chair slightly higher than yours. If you want them to feel vulnerable, direct them to a chair lower than yours.

EYE CONTACT Part of a show of personal interest is an intent gaze focused on your partner's eyes. This makes the person feel special since research has shown that sexual interest is demonstrated by enlargement of the pupils and that this, in itself, is arousing. Men and women, judging photographs where one of a pair has had the pupils of the eyes enlarged by retouching, always rated that picture as the more attractive. (But don't overdo the gazing, or you will just look silly.)

EMULATION Body language can be used to emulate that of a person you are talking to, and reinforces the sense of matching. When a person shifts position, you can copy that shift. Once tuned in to the other person's body movements you can start altering your own, slowly, so that your body becomes open and receptive. The object of your attentions is likely to copy you unconsciously and assimilate the new feeling of intimacy this creates.

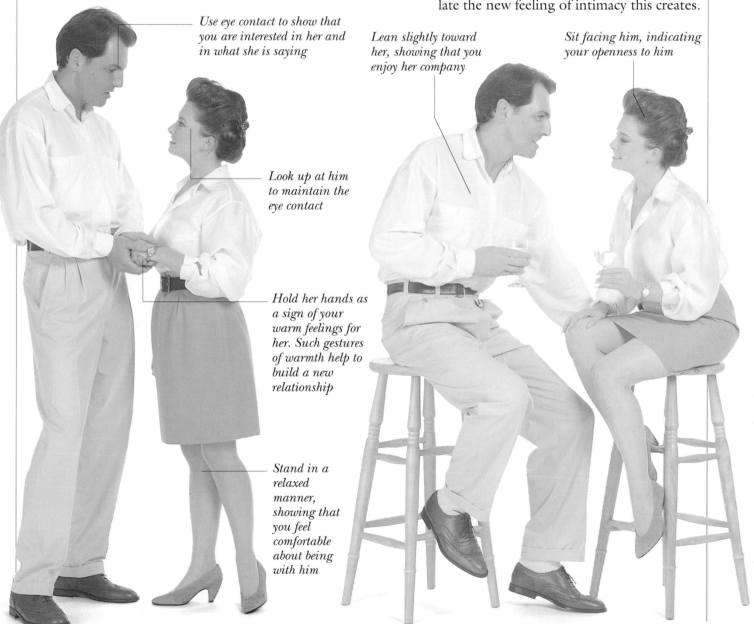

Use eye contact to show that you are interested in her and in what she is saying

Look up at him to maintain the eye contact

Hold her hands as a sign of your warm feelings for her. Such gestures of warmth help to build a new relationship

Stand in a relaxed manner, showing that you feel comfortable about being with him

Lean slightly toward her, showing that you enjoy her company

Sit facing him, indicating your openness to him

Stage 3 USE TOUCH TO SUGGEST INTIMACY

There are a number of occasions and opportunities when you can indulge in deliberate touches that charge your meetings with eroticism. It is important, though, that you deliberately hold back for a while from anything overtly sexual so that you lay the groundwork for a buildup of sexual tension: a mild withdrawal can seem tantalizingly provoking. Because your behavior will create mild anxiety, your partner's entire arousal level will be raised, thus readying him or her to be erotically receptive.

CONVEY WARMTH Hold hands on introduction a little longer than necessary. Look directly into your friend's eyes while talking, but don't stare at them. Use touch to convey warmth; for example, when you feel good about something give him or her a hug. If you feel concerned about something that the other is worried about, display your sympathy by covering his or her hand with yours. When walking, demonstrate your concern for that person's well-being by slipping your hand under his or her arm.

If you accompany a friend to a party or dance where you are standing together much of the time, stand close. When you are in crowds, put a protective arm around him or her.

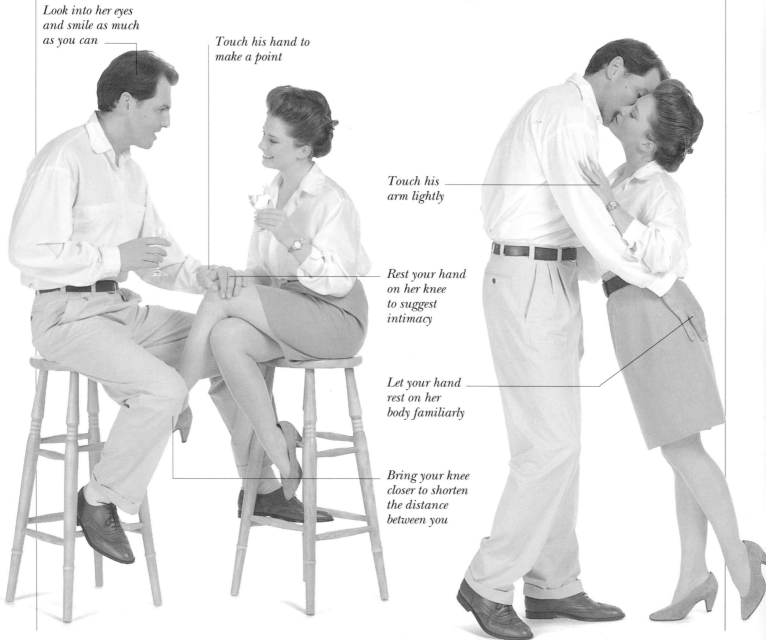

Look into her eyes and smile as much as you can

Touch his hand to make a point

Touch his arm lightly

Rest your hand on her knee to suggest intimacy

Let your hand rest on her body familiarly

Bring your knee closer to shorten the distance between you

INTRIGUING TOUCH As you get to know each other more, put an arm around your partner as you walk, and instead of resting a hand on his or her waist, place it farther down the side of the hip. If your hand reaches around near the pubis, even though this is still a casual touch, it begins to feel suggestive to the person experiencing it. But because they don't know whether or not you mean it suggestively, it also becomes intriguing. A variation on this move is to rest your hand on your partner's waist, and then let it slip a little lower so that it is on the small of the back or even resting on the top of the buttocks.

KISSING Kiss as a greeting: kiss your partner lightly at first, but as time goes by and you get to know each other better, make the kiss more direct and more lingering. Don't oblit-

erate your partner with the first kiss; make it light and exploratory, rather than fevered and oppressive. This may sound like very basic advice, but by following it you are setting the scene for truly sensual lovemaking.

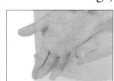

Sensual erotic touch p28

By creating unhurried but sensual beginnings, in which your partner receives a sense of choice without feeling pressured, you are creating important foundations upon which to build a happy and successful sexual relationship. And when you get to know your partner better, and you begin to spend more time alone together, you will find that you have many opportunities to make everyday situations more sensual by the use of erotic touch. This will build up the sense of intimacy between you and deepen the feelings you have for each other.

IMPROVING YOUR APPEARANCE

POINTERS FOR MEN

- **FACIAL APPEARANCE** If you have a beard, consider altering the shape of it to allow your more sensual facial features, such as your lips and cheekbones, to show through more clearly. Your hair should, of course, be clean and neat, but it may also benefit from trimming or even a total restyling, preferably by a good hairdresser.

- **GLASSES** If you wear glasses, are they as flattering to your facial shape as possible? If not, invest in some that are — the range of frame shapes and colors now available means that practically everyone can find a style that suits them. Or consider a change to contact lenses.

- **UNDERWEAR** Many women prefer the appearance of boxer shorts to that of briefs, but whatever your personal preference is, the important thing is that they should be clean and a good fit. Old-fashioned cotton undershirts may be practical, but the new colored underwear that clings suggestively to the form is sexier.

- **CLOTHES** Stylish casual clothes, starting with basic jackets and trousers, can slowly be acquired to replace old drab garments. Beware of bright colors, if you wouldn't normally wear them, but concentrate your attention on the style and cut of your clothes: for example, blouson-style jackets team well with classic jeans or with casual trousers. If you are plump, beware of buying trousers that are pleated in front. Trousers with straight panels at the waist invariably look slim and sexy.

POINTERS FOR WOMEN

- **FACIAL APPEARANCE** Emphasize your facial features to bring out the best in them — outline your eyes and lips to accentuate them, and highlight your cheek contours with blusher. Pay attention to your hair; have it cut or restyled if it doesn't become you the way it is, and if it is a dull color, brighten or tint it. Don't forget to adapt the shades of your makeup to match your new hair tones.

- **GLASSES** If you wear glasses, are they as flattering to your facial shape as possible? If they are not, invest in some with frames that are a better shape or color, or consider a change to contact lenses.

- **UNDERWEAR** Throw away old-fashioned, boring underwear and invest in lacy briefs, bras, and teddies — knowing that you are wearing sexy underwear, and the sensation of it against your skin, will make you feel sexier and more self-confident. Wear discreetly patterned hose that show off the shape of your legs, and alternate these with lacy garter belts and sheer stockings.

- **SHOES** Start buying shoes with higher heels than you normally wear.

- **CLOTHES** Invest in dresses, skirts, and pants that cling and are made of sensual materials. Focus gradually on showing off the shape of your body.

- **SCENT** When you take a shower or bath, use body lotions and spend time selecting a light but fragrant perfume that enhances your natural scents.

SENSUAL EROTIC TOUCH

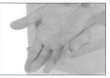

A variety of situations, including casual everyday experiences, can become more sensual and erotic by the use of deliberate touch. Close body contact and gentle movements will not only relax your partner, but make him or her aware of your presence at a level deeper than conscious sensation.

BRUSH YOUR PARTNER'S HAIR Brush away from the forehead toward the back of the head, first with your fingertips and then with a hairbrush.

Use a bristle hairbrush to stimulate the scalp, taking care not to pull or tangle the hair

START FROM THE TOP Nestle close to your partner and, with your thumbs, knead the muscles at the base of the neck and across the shoulders.

MASSAGE THE SCALP Work those massaging fingers up the neck and into the scalp. Give a gentle scalp massage with your fingertips by separately rotating the scalp, and then the hair, in tiny circles.

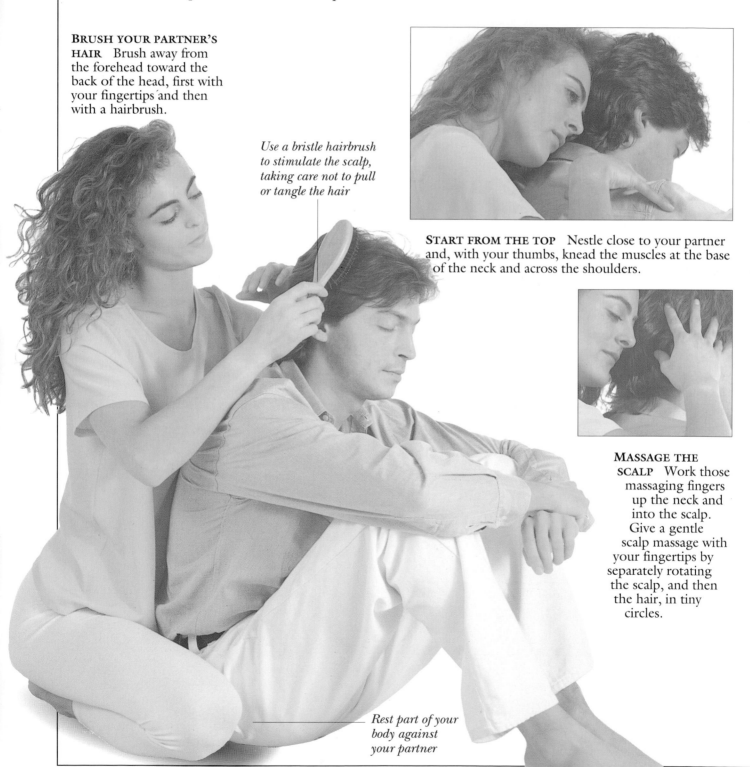

Rest part of your body against your partner

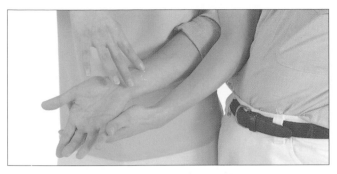

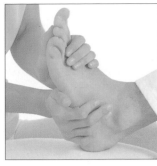

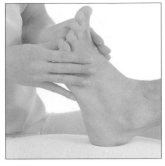

TRAIL YOUR NAILS ALONG THE ARMS Lightly draw your fingernails from the crook of the elbow down to the wrist. Repeat this several times in different areas of the inner arms.

MASSAGE THE SOLES With both hands, and with thumb and forefinger, then your whole hand, massage the sole of each foot with a circling movement.

WORK ON THE TOES Gently push a slippery forefinger in and out between each of your partner's toes, turning it from side to side.

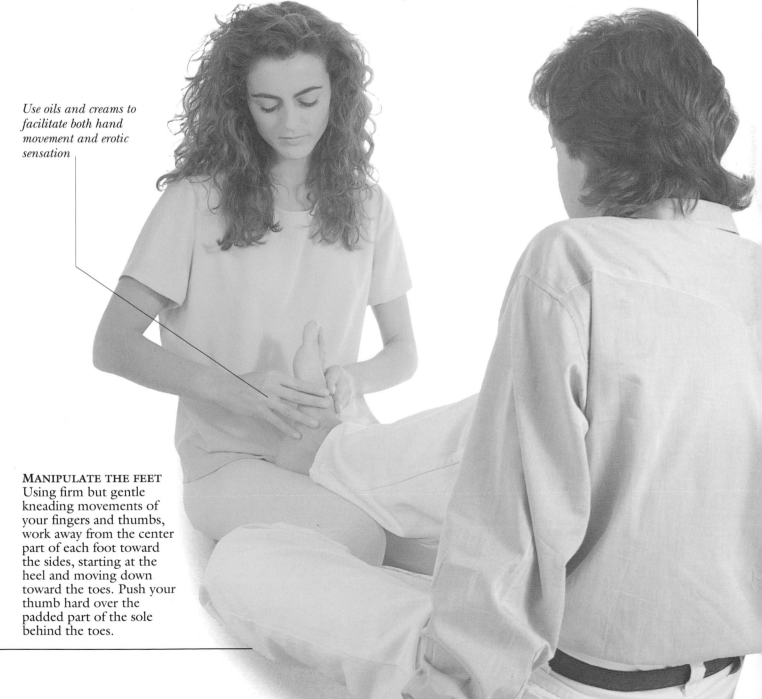

Use oils and creams to facilitate both hand movement and erotic sensation

MANIPULATE THE FEET Using firm but gentle kneading movements of your fingers and thumbs, work away from the center part of each foot toward the sides, starting at the heel and moving down toward the toes. Push your thumb hard over the padded part of the sole behind the toes.

BASIC LOVEMAKING POSITIONS

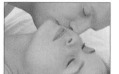 *There are many different positions in which you can make love, and these simple and straightforward ones are generally recommended when starting a new relationship. They offer opportunities for intimacy as well as satisfying each partner's need to take control. However, because it is possible to make love in so many ways, trying new positions can be fun and will help keep your lovemaking from settling into a predictable routine — which can lead to the boredom that often destroys relationships.*

THE MISSIONARY POSITION   The missionary is so called because, allegedly, missionaries sent out to "civilize" the colonies of the old European empires thought that it was the only respectable position for decent people, and insisted that their new converts use it when making love. Despite its staid image, however, it is an enjoyable position with many variations.

You should support your weight on one or both of your hands or elbows to make the most of this position

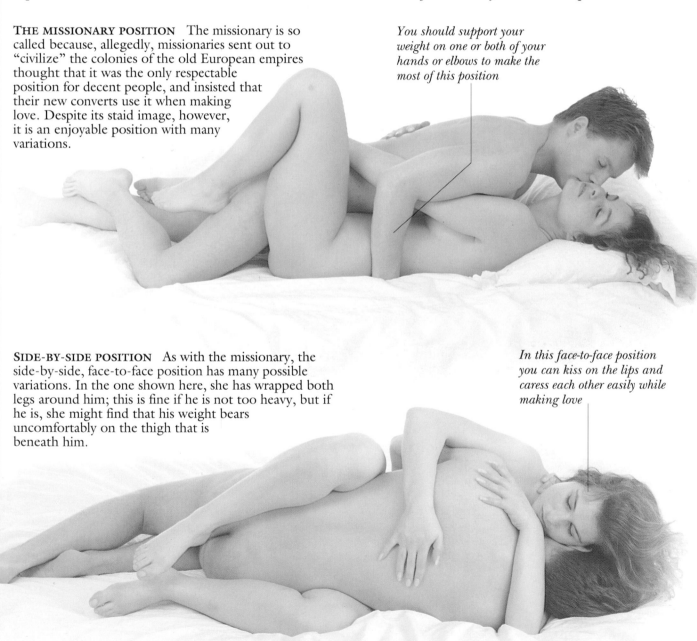

SIDE-BY-SIDE POSITION   As with the missionary, the side-by-side, face-to-face position has many possible variations. In the one shown here, she has wrapped both legs around him; this is fine if he is not too heavy, but if he is, she might find that his weight bears uncomfortably on the thigh that is beneath him.

In this face-to-face position you can kiss on the lips and caress each other easily while making love

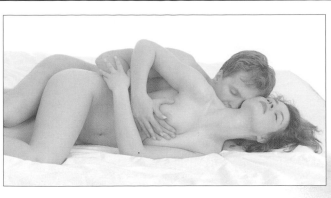

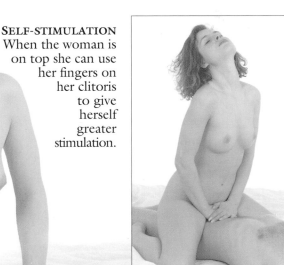

You can use your fingers and hands to stroke and stimulate your partner's genitals and other erogenous zones

THE SPOONS POSITION The spoons is a rear-entry position in which the couple snuggles up together, forming a shape said to be like a pair of spoons nestled together. Pleasant variations on this position include her pushing one leg back between his after penetration; him leaning backward away from her; and her bending forward from the waist. The last two variations usually allow greater penetration.

When you are on top, you can control the movements and the depth of penetration

REAR ENTRY There are many rear-entry positions besides the spoons and its variations. These include the well-known kneeling (or "doggy") position shown here, as well as standing, lying, and sitting positions, and those where she sits astride and facing away from him.

WOMAN ON TOP There are many different woman-on-top variations. For instance, she can kneel astride him and then sit upright; lean forward or lean backward; she can lie on top of him with her legs outside his or between them; or he can sit up with her on his lap.

SELF-STIMULATION When the woman is on top she can use her fingers on her clitoris to give herself greater stimulation.

As well as being able to stimulate yourself, you can use your hands to give your partner extra stimulation too

31

HOW CAN I TUNE IN TO WHAT MY PARTNER WANTS?

"There is no harm in saying to your partner, on hearing the question 'What do you like?' the words, 'I'm not really sure but I'd certainly love the chance to find out.' After all, it gives both of you glorious carte blanche."

MANY A MAN subscribes to the myth that he ought to know everything about his woman's sexual needs and that he should be able to read her mind. This is left over from the time when the male was traditionally expected to be active in the sexual relationship and the woman passive. And many women suffer from not knowing what it is their male partners would like. These worries can be an especially heavy load if you don't happen to be sexually experienced.

In addition, there are nearly always situations when we feel uncomfortable. New ideas about men's and women's changing roles question sexual as well as social values and place us in situations our upbringing has not equipped us for. For example, a man, dining with a woman friend, may find it hard to cope if she propositions him directly. He may not know how to respond, because she will have stepped outside an age-old formula of dating and mating. If he says yes, does that mean he is somehow too easy and therefore weak? If he says no, will he seem like a prude, or a coward who can't deal with the modern woman?

CASE STUDY *Jon & Nora*

Jon and Nora were both sexually inexperienced, and neither knew how to go about finding out what their partners enjoyed. Jon thought that asking for sexual information would reflect badly on him while Nora asked, rightly, how you can become experienced without being sexual in the first place.

Name:	JON
Age:	24
Marital status:	SINGLE
Occupation:	SOUND ENGINEER

Jon was tall, slim, and blond, and full of nervous energy that made him very extroverted yet inwardly anxious where forming new sexual relationships was concerned.

"I want a girlfriend to love me so much," he said. "I'm dying to wake up in the morning with someone's arms around me, and to feel love for her and know she cares about me. For me, falling in love and making a relationship are based on sex. If the sex part of the relationship isn't right, then I can't love someone.

"The two women I really cared for dumped me, not vice versa. That means I'm feeling very uncertain of myself. I'm just getting into a new relationship, but now I'm scared that I'm somehow going to miss what she really wants, both from the relationship and from sex. How can I find out what my partner really wants?"

Name:	NORA
Age:	29
Marital status:	SINGLE
Occupation:	WORD PROCESSOR

Nora had almost waist-length blond hair, and because she was so beautifully groomed she looked like a model. Yet she was, in fact, shy and retiring, having lived all her life in her parents' home. She had only had one lover, a colleague by the name of Bobby.

"I know I've got a lot to learn sexually," she told me. "I never had an orgasm with Bobby, and he used to tell me I was full of inhibitions and probably frigid. I'm not frigid because I can have orgasms on my own, through masturbation, but when I meet a new man who interests me — and there's one on the scene now — I get confused.

"I'm honestly not sure what I want from him. Getting on his wavelength seems fraught with difficulty. He keeps asking me how I like to make love. The trouble is, I don't really know. But you feel like such a wimp saying that. How can I find out what I want without making love with him in the first place? And what happens if I want things he doesn't seem to be offering? I want to please him. How can I reply when he asks me what I want?"

THERAPIST'S ASSESSMENT

Jon was worried that asking his new partner what she wanted in their lovemaking would reveal his inexperience and make him seem unattractive. In reality, by enquiring about his partner's likes and dislikes, Jon would be showing that he was interested in her as an individual, and not as a sexual machine off an assembly line.

ASKING QUESTIONS
One way of getting comfortable with asking sexual questions is to think through a phase of lovemaking in your mind. For example, if a man in Jon's situation wants to know if his lover really enjoys her breasts being touched, before he actually asks her he can imagine himself lying naked in bed with her in his arms. In his thoughts, he slowly runs his fingers around her breasts, gently pinching and rubbing her nipples a little. As he does so he says to her, "Does that feel good?" Then, running his fingertips along the sides of her breasts from her armpits down to the bottom, he asks, "Or does this feel better?" By giving her options for her answer he is less likely to bulldoze her into saying it was good when it wasn't. He will also provide himself with accurate information. Going from there, in his fantasy, he could say to her, "I'd like it if you would tell me if I do anything you dislike."

I suggested that Jon rehearse such scenes mentally, so that the real event would be much easier to handle. Then both he and his woman friend would feel more confident about discussing their likes and dislikes.

FINDING OUT WHAT YOU PREFER
Nora's problem lay in finding out what she would like, so that she could tell her partner about it. Once again, I recommended rehearsing various sexual situations mentally — in Nora's case, to enable her to predict the emotions that such situations would arouse in her if they happened in real life.

We all experience a variety of reactions when considering these situations, such as arousal, discomfort, or dislike. Arousal and dislike speak for themselves. Discomfort, however, does not indicate unsuitability of, but rather unfamiliarity with, an activity we might like to try. We feel discomfort when we are faced with something new that we are unprepared for. Rehearsing some of these scenes will help give you confidence should you find yourself choosing one of them in reality.

My program for IMPROVING SEXUAL COMMUNICATION

This program is intended to make both partners in a relationship aware of each other's sexual likes and needs. Discussing and actually demonstrating sexual proclivities is essential for a relationship to succeed. Don't worry if you feel inhibited or embarrassed at first, or if your partner does. If you each mentally rehearse the parts that you find awkward, and then take those rehearsals into real life, you will end up knowing a great deal about your partner's erotic responses. You will also have knocked down walls of inhibition, fostering an invaluable intimacy between you. Like all the best therapy exercises, however, this program for improving sexual communication is deceptively simple.

Stage I INITIATING COMMUNICATION

It is just as important for your partner to know what you like as it is for you to know what your partner likes. But not all of us are good at expressing our likes and dislikes in words, and some of us find it especially difficult to express feelings and desires about lovemaking. Sometimes, therefore, the part-

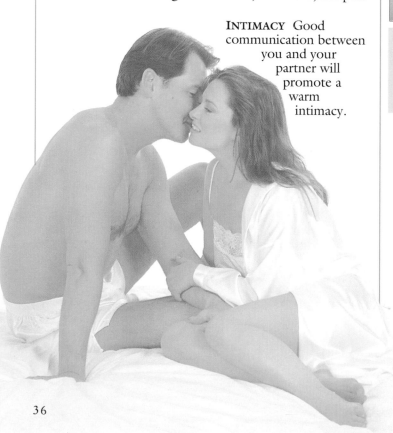

INTIMACY Good communication between you and your partner will promote a warm intimacy.

ners in a relationship find that communication about sexual likes is best done with actions and demonstrations as well as through conversation.

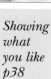

Showing what you like p38

TAKE TURNS If that is the case for you or your partner, you might find it useful to take turns demonstrating what each of you likes, sharing the experience as much as possible. Even if you are both quite happy to discuss your sexual needs and desires, you might still find it useful (as well as pleasurable) to demonstrate to each other what it is that you like to do or have done to you.

SEXUAL AWARENESS Of course, you may not be sure exactly what it is that you want from sex, or you may know what you want but find it hard to discuss the subject. This often happens when we are sexually inexperienced and relatively unaware of our own sexual responses, and it is something that happens to us all when we first become sexually active.

Many people find that a program of self-pleasuring (see pages 226 and 228) helps them to develop an awareness of their own sexual responses, and that this awareness provides them with useful knowledge to bring to their sexual relationships.

And if you are shy about discussing such intimately personal matters as your sexual preferences, the sexual assertiveness program on page 72 will show you how to overcome your reticence so that you can discuss your sexual likes and dislikes openly.

Stage 2 SHARING A SEXUAL BIOGRAPHY

One of the results of living in a culture where discussions about sex are still partly taboo is that we do not normally share sexual information about ourselves. But even when we are willing to disclose such information, some of us don't consider ourselves to have been particularly sexual in the past, and so feel that we have little to say on the subject. Yet we are all sexual beings from the minute we are born, and our very earliest experiences have a bearing on how we relate to a partner in the here and now.

Thinking back to our early days, asking ourselves a few pertinent questions, and then sharing the information with a new partner, is a wonderful way to give that partner a full picture of who we are today. Even if you have never been to bed with anyone, it is still possible to work out, from life experience, just what is going to matter to you (and therefore to your new lover).

The questionnaire on the right is designed to stimulate your sexual memories. Set aside periods of time in which you can talk through these memories with your partner, and corresponding periods for your partner to talk through his or her memories with you. You will need at least a couple of hours each. If you turn out to be really interested and interesting, the sex talk could go on for days.

MEMORIES Sharing sexual memories with your partner helps you get to know each other better.

SEXUAL BIOGRAPHY QUESTIONNAIRE

• What was your parents' background? What was their occupation, religion and culture?

• What were their moral attitudes and their views on enjoyment and play?

• Were your parents affectionate toward each other, or were they tense and aggressive toward each other?

• What do you remember of incidents that may relate to your parents' sex life?

• What was their attitude toward nudity?

• Looking back, how successful would you rate your parents' marriage, both sexually and socially?

• What kind of hidden messages do you think you received from your parents with regard to sex?

• What kind of attitudes to sex do you think you acquired during childhood?

• When and how did you first learn about sex?

• Were there any early sexual experiences that were embarrassing or humiliating for you?

• When did you first masturbate?

• Do you have sexual fantasies? And, if so, at what age did they begin?

• Did you or do you have crushes on people of the same sex?

• If you are a man, at what age did you first have wet dreams? If you are a woman, at what age did you start menstruation?

• What was your earliest sexual experience? Was it with someone of the same sex as you, or someone of the opposite sex?

• What have your subsequent sexual experiences and relationships been like?

37

DEMONSTRATING
WHAT YOU LIKE

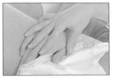

Unless your partner knows what you like or how you become aroused, you can easily be turned off sexually. Demonstration is often the best way of communicating. Take turns stimulating yourselves and touching each other's pleasurable areas, so that each of you shows the other what really turns you on. Encourage your partner when he or she is doing something that is particularly arousing for you.

DEMONSTRATE EROGENOUS ZONES
Put your hand over your partner's while you are being caressed, and guide it to your favorite erogenous zones. These might include — apart from your genitals — your nipples, the insides of your thighs, your perineum and your anus, and any other area of your body that, when touched or stroked, arouses you sexually.

Watch your partner's reactions to being touched in a certain spot; this will tell you a lot about its sensitivity

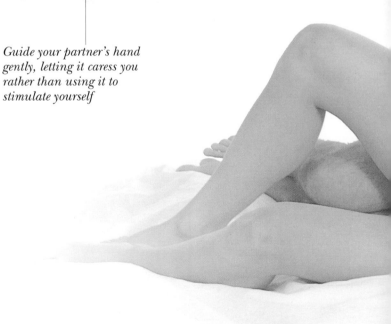

Guide your partner's hand gently, letting it caress you rather than using it to stimulate yourself

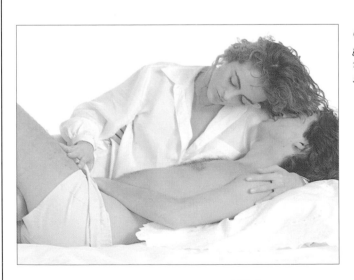

DEMONSTRATE SELF-STIMULATION While your partner watches, demonstrate how you like to caress yourself. Explain what you do and how it feels, and include all your favorite erogenous zones.

HAND-ON-HAND STIMULATION With your partner's hand lightly covering the back of yours, caress, stroke and stimulate yourself. Show your partner how best to touch and arouse you, and demonstrate the kind of pressure, motion and rhythm that is most effective. Describe your preferences; for example, say if you prefer your nipples to be stimulated by gentle massage of the tips or by having a fingertip circle the sides.

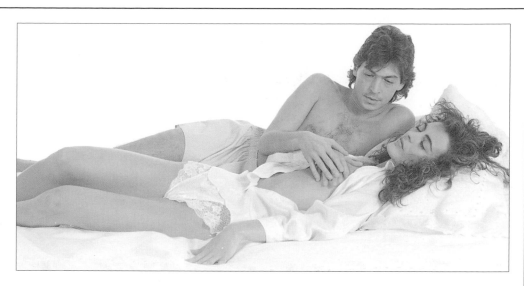

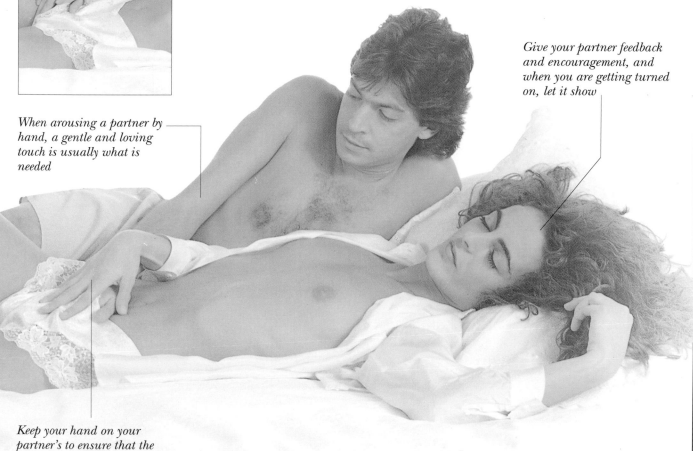

GUIDE YOUR PARTNER Take hold of your partner's hand and use it as you would your own to stimulate your genitals and the area around them, including your pubic region, the insides of your thighs and your perineum.

LET YOUR PARTNER STIMULATE YOU When you have shown where your erogenous zones are and how you like them to be touched, let your partner stimulate them. Keep a hand lightly on your partner's, so that you can supply any guidance that might be necessary, but let your partner do the actual stimulation and so learn how best to turn you on.

Give your partner feedback and encouragement, and when you are getting turned on, let it show

When arousing a partner by hand, a gentle and loving touch is usually what is needed

Keep your hand on your partner's to ensure that the right areas are stimulated

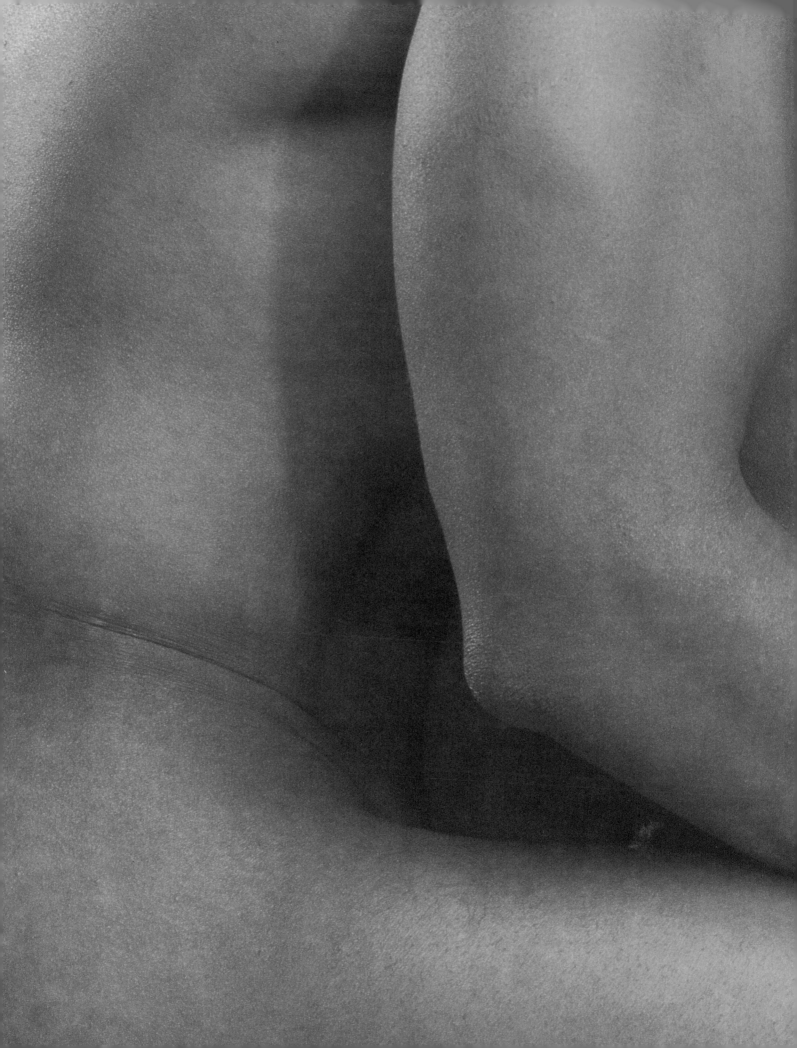

CHAPTER 3

HOW CAN I OVERCOME MY PARTNER'S INHIBIT~ IONS?

"You can strike a blow for your generation's sexual freedom in the privacy of your own bedroom."

MANY PEOPLE COME to me because they feel inhibited in their sexual responses. Often this problem is a result of difficult personal experiences that they have had at some time in the past, or of their being influenced too greatly by societal attitudes. But sometimes the cause of the problem is simply that the individuals involved are being rushed by their partners.

Personal counseling can help when family members or other inhibiting persons are creating problems, and it is important that we recognize that some inhibitions stem from attitudes in society that have been handed down from generation to generation to keep control of our sexual behavior.

However, if a person's sexual inhibitions are the result of feeling rushed, the guidelines in my program can be used by everyone to combat this. Personal sexual exploration, for example, which teaches individuals about their own sexual response patterns and, equally importantly, how to enjoy sexual pleasure without feeling guilty, is often a great help in dealing with inhibitions.

CASE STUDY *Louis & Charlotte*

Charlotte's sexual inhibitions, largely the result of the influence of her domineering and moralistic father, were aggravated by the impatience of her partner, Louis. Charlotte wanted to shed her inhibitions, and in order to help her Louis had to learn to take life at a gentler pace.

Name:	LOUIS
Age:	29
Marital status:	SINGLE
Occupation:	STOCKBROKER

Louis was a busy young professional. Wearing a well-tailored suit and complete with a cellular phone, he gave the impression of being in a continual rush.

"I've been dating Charlotte for a month and find her very attractive," he told me. "She is gorgeous to look at and extremely bright. Frankly, because of that I expected her to be hot stuff in bed. Maybe she is. I don't know. She never has been when she's with me.

"I've rarely met a woman so inhibited. When we make love she just lies there, completely frozen. But she is obviously attracted to me, because when we're not in a sexual situation she winds herself around me and she seems to be tremendously turned on. What I want to know is this: is there really any point in us continuing with the relationship if the sexual side isn't working?"

Name:	CHARLOTTE
Age:	25
Marital status:	SINGLE
Occupation:	LIBRARIAN

Charlotte had huge, dark eyes, bouncy black curls, and an engaging, lively personality. Her entire appearance seemed seductive, yet when she talked about her difficulty in making sexual relationships her confidence deserted her, and she rapidly became distressed.

"I'm only really attracted to high-powered men," she confessed. "But I know I need a lot of time to unwind sexually, and businessmen like Louis rarely have that to spare. I can already sense his impatience with me. I've only had two other serious love affairs. Neither lasted more than a year, and only one of them really worked sexually. Even then I didn't have a climax. I know I need time to relax and get to know someone before I can start to be sexual. How can I get Louis to take things more slowly?

"My father was strictly religious and extremely moral, and although I don't agree with his views on sex, I do find myself remembering them at the most inconvenient times. In fact, as soon as I find myself in a sexual situation, I actually feel that I can see his face looking at me."

THERAPIST'S ASSESSMENT

Charlotte was a textbook case of someone trying to live up to her difficult and demanding father all over again in her adult life — only for "father," read "lover." Trained by her father's volatile temper, she was continually tense and awaiting impatient explosion, so it was hardly surprising that she couldn't relax with Louis, who barely disguised his need to get her cured quickly. Charlotte had a double burden because she had also taken in, on a deep level, binding moral messages, so much so that when she found herself getting turned on she instantly imagined her father's face judging her.

PERSONAL SEXUAL EXPLORATION

Charlotte needed to do some personal work, with a therapist, on understanding the effect her father had had on her. This helped her to substitute pleasurable mental images for thoughts of her inhibiting father. She also needed to do some personal sexual exploration of herself (page 232) since she revealed that not only had she never experienced climax, she also had never attempted masturbation. Finding out about her sexuality, discovering its pleasures and the fact that retribution did not fall on her if she enjoyed it, went a long way toward improving her chances with a man.

Whether Louis is the right lover for her remains to be seen. Unless he can learn to change his rushed behavior, he probably isn't. But the fact that he was willing to seek help was a positive sign and meant that it was certainly worth the couple trying a sexual enhancement program together (page 60).

SEXUAL ENHANCEMENT

Louis also needed some help, because he saw women as objects to consume or to smooth his life in his rush for the top of the career ladder. What he hadn't yet worked out for himself was the fact that haste has its price. In his case, the price was that of immense pressure, a sense that he had to carry everything and everybody on his shoulders, Charlotte's sex problem included. Through practicing joint sexual enhancement exercises together with Charlotte, Louis learned that she was an individual with responsibility for herself, rather than a personal burden. He also received the opportunity to create spaces in his life in which to relax, calm down, and enjoy himself.

My program for
LOSING INHIBITIONS

There are many factors that can affect mental and physical sexual expression. Tension, for example, is a component of sexual response, but too much of it can block excitement and arousal. Sexual repression is another inhibitor of successful lovemaking, and many of us are embarrassed by sex. We find it hard to let go, fearing we will appear primitive or animalistic if we give vent to cries or spontaneous sexual movements. Spending time discovering what makes us feel good, and being able to express those feelings, will make our sexual experiences more satisfying.

Stage 1 PROJECT A SEXIER IMAGE

If you look inhibited, you will probably feel inhibited, and thus narrow your opportunities for joyful sexual expression. By making changes in your outward appearance so that you project a sexier image (see pages 24-27), you can begin to alter your inner responses.

LEARN TO RELAX
Relaxation exercises can help to dispel the tension that often fuels inhibitions.

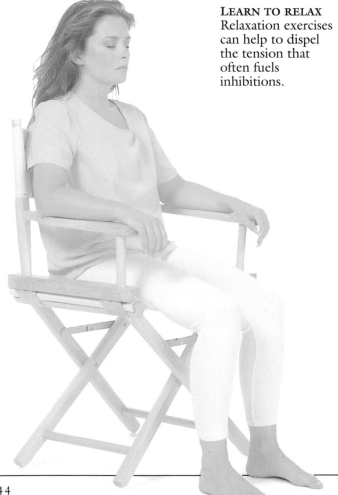

Stage 2 USE RELAXATION EXERCISES

Deliberately practicing relaxation exercises before lovemaking can dispel tension and make the difference between eroticism and despair. Neither partner should feel rushed to respond, and being relaxed means that you can more quickly attune yourself with not only what your partner finds pleasurable but also what you are experiencing.

As a general rule, relaxation exercises are best carried out lying flat on your back. But because this may not always be practical, the relaxation exercises that are described in the box on the facing page have been chosen because they can be practiced in a sitting position, in a comfortable chair.

PREPARATION Before you begin your relaxation exercises, prepare your surroundings. Make sure that you are not going to be disturbed and that the room is warm and comfortable. Then, as a prelude to your relaxation exercises, take a long, warm bath, which will help you to relax.

Stage 3 GIVE VENT TO SEXUAL EXPRESSION

An effective way to keep in tune with your sexual responses is to practice self-pleasuring routines (see pages 226-229). Give yourself an hour of privacy, and relax on your bed in a warm room. Caress your body where you know it feels good, moving down toward your genitals. If you usually lie on your back when you masturbate, try it from some other position, such as lying on your side.

RESPOND TO YOUR AROUSAL Let out gasps of breath and make yourself moan when you begin to feel aroused. Try moving your legs around and stroke the rest of your body with the hand that isn't massaging your genitals. Start off by making slow body movements, but deliberately exaggerate them as you become aroused, and move your pubis against your fingers so that your whole body is active.

As you get aroused, practice saying a few sexual words, quietly but deliberately. As you near orgasm allow your breathing to sound in the room, let yourself gasp and sigh, allow those breaths to become heavier and louder. If you want to scream when you reach orgasm, don't stifle it — let go.

Self-stimulation p230

EXAMINE YOUR FEELINGS If there are aspects of this exercise that make you embarrassed or ashamed, think back into your family history. Where did those attitudes come from? Practice the exercise again a few days later, and compare the moments that embarrassed you the first time with what discomfited you the second time. Are they different? Are you growing more comfortable with noise and movement? As you survive the uncomfortable moments, is it getting a little easier to do the exercise? It's important to practice this somewhat exaggerated behavior slowly, and you may need to do the exercise at least twice a week for some time before you really feel comfortable about it.

Stage 4 DRESS TO STIMULATE EROTIC TOUCH

At the beginning of a sexual relationship we often feel hesitant about taking our clothes off. Meeting up with a partner who actually enjoys making love while clothed not only can be a relief to the inhibited, it can be deliberately piquant to those people who would normally only make love when naked. Erotic touch, combined with sensual clothing, very definitely enhances lovemaking. The ways of doing this are as varied as is the imagination and the wardrobe. For instance, a woman could play the temptress — while wearing a cat suit and refusing to take it off, she could strip her partner and use her hands and her clothed body to stimulate his naked skin. Then she could either leave him aroused but unfulfilled, promising intercourse later, or strip and make love to him.

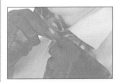

Playing the temptress p46

RELAXATION EXERCISES

This simple but effective relaxation exercise routine includes deep breathing, mental relaxation, and an exercise to release the muscular tension from your body. As well as using these exercises as a prelude to exploring your own sexual responses, you can practice them whenever you want to relax and unwind, for instance, at the end of a busy day.

• **HEEL PRESSURE** Sit on a firm but comfortable chair with your feet about a foot apart from each other on the floor, and push down with your heels for a count of ten. As you do so, enjoy the feeling of being connected to the ground through your heels. When you stop pushing down with your heels, try to retain that feeling of connectedness with the ground. Then start to pay attention to your breathing — get into a steady rhythm of breathing in slowly through your nose and letting go through your mouth.

• **DEEP BREATHING** To begin with, you will probably be breathing shallowly from the chest. But as you continue, grow aware of your breathing moving deeper within your body until it is originating from the diaphragm. Once you have reached what feels like a comfortable rhythm, continue automatically while concentrating on your thoughts.

• **THOUGHTS** Close your eyes and try to focus your thoughts on one thing, such as a tiny, imaginary pinpoint of light in the darkness. Let your body relax into the most comfortable sitting position you can find, and clear your mind of any intrusive thoughts that may arise (this will become easier after a few sessions, when you no longer have to give much thought to what you are supposed to be doing next in the routine).

• **TENSE AND RELAX** Pay attention to your limbs: some of them may remain tense. Starting with your left foot, deliberately clench it in as tight a muscle spasm as you can manage. Hold this for a count of five and then let go. Repeat the tense-and-relax routine with your whole left leg, your right foot and right leg, and then your buttocks, first one side and then the other, then both together. Give your stomach, shoulders, left hand, left arm, right hand and right arm the same treatment, and then screw up your face for a count of five.

• **RELEASING TENSION** By exaggerating the tension and then letting it go, you end up ridding your body of tension completely. Spend fifteen minutes on working through your body, searching out the trouble spots and applying the tense-and-relax pattern. Once you feel relaxed, sit back and enjoy the lack of tension for a while, perhaps for an extra five or ten minutes if circumstances allow.

PLAYING THE TEMPTRESS

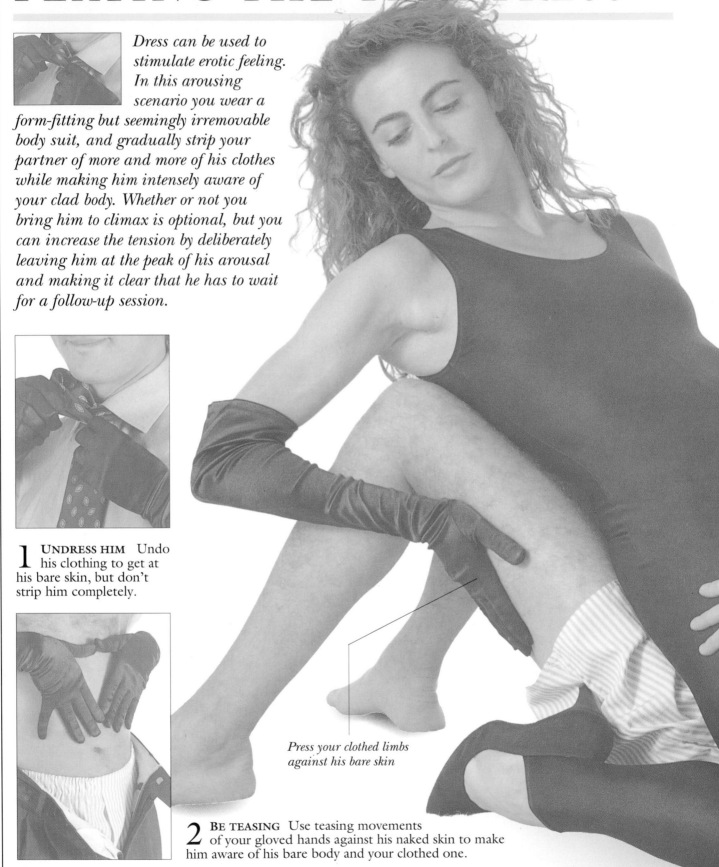

Dress can be used to stimulate erotic feeling. In this arousing scenario you wear a form-fitting but seemingly irremovable body suit, and gradually strip your partner of more and more of his clothes while making him intensely aware of your clad body. Whether or not you bring him to climax is optional, but you can increase the tension by deliberately leaving him at the peak of his arousal and making it clear that he has to wait for a follow-up session.

1 UNDRESS HIM Undo his clothing to get at his bare skin, but don't strip him completely.

2 BE TEASING Use teasing movements of your gloved hands against his naked skin to make him aware of his bare body and your clothed one.

Press your clothed limbs against his bare skin

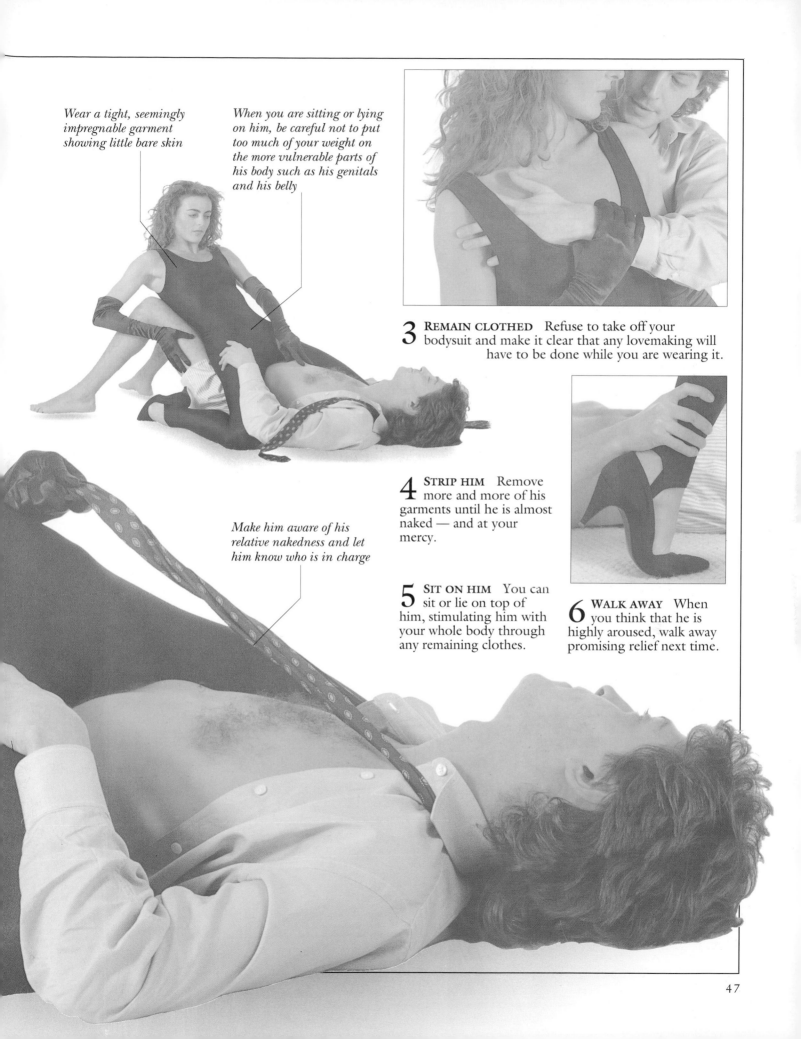

Wear a tight, seemingly impregnable garment showing little bare skin

When you are sitting or lying on him, be careful not to put too much of your weight on the more vulnerable parts of his body such as his genitals and his belly

3 **REMAIN CLOTHED** Refuse to take off your bodysuit and make it clear that any lovemaking will have to be done while you are wearing it.

4 **STRIP HIM** Remove more and more of his garments until he is almost naked — and at your mercy.

Make him aware of his relative nakedness and let him know who is in charge

5 **SIT ON HIM** You can sit or lie on top of him, stimulating him with your whole body through any remaining clothes.

6 **WALK AWAY** When you think that he is highly aroused, walk away promising relief next time.

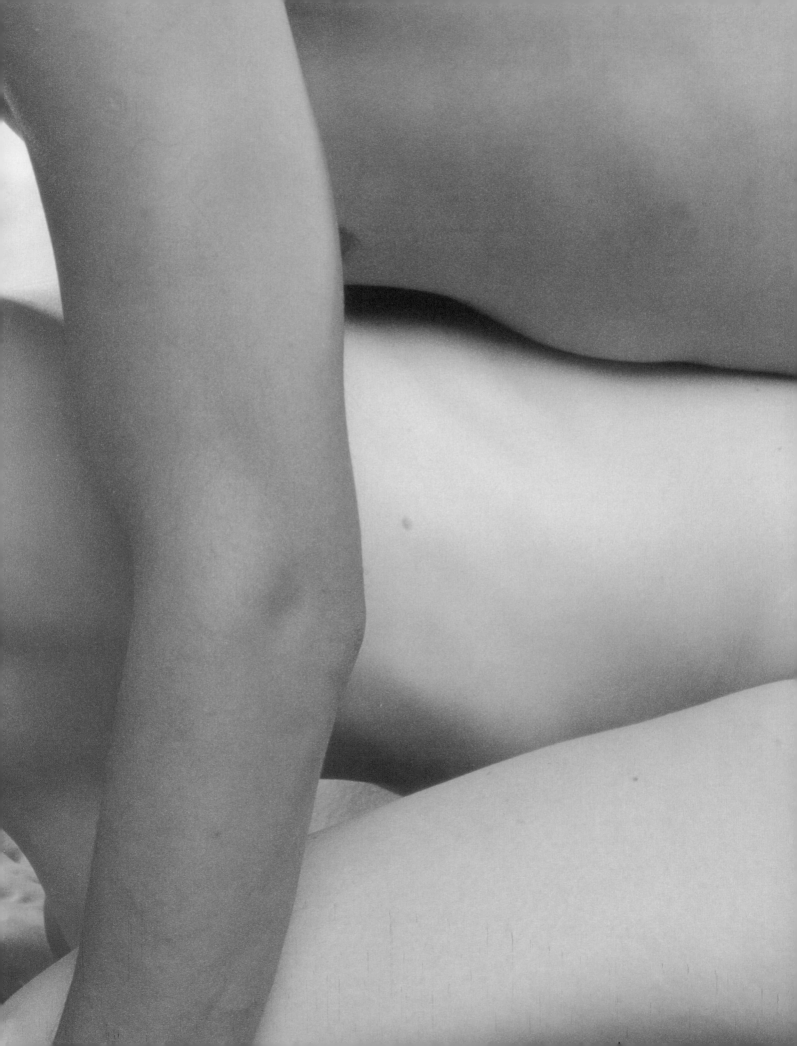

CHAPTER 4

HOW CAN I FULLY AROUSE MY PARTNER?

"Since good sex was always supposed to be spontaneous, it has been unacceptable to consider the idea of planning. And yet, if we truly want to increase our sexual options, that's what we need to do."

HOWEVER DIFFICULT a relationship may have been, men and women grow accustomed to the pattern of certain activities. Lovemaking is a prime example. It is possible to have sex with a husband or wife, year in and year out, with very little love involved, and yet the mechanics of the sex act will work perfectly.

Take away the feeling of familiarity, substitute a new partner, and a load of insecurities rear their insinuating heads in the subconscious. Sometimes it simply feels wrong to be making love to another, however irrational you know that feeling to be. Sometimes it is the pattern of lovemaking itself that traps you. Only the old one will work, but the partner who provided it is no longer in your life.

Sometimes the problem is one of trust; you can't fully trust somebody until they have fulfilled certain psychological criteria. Within lovemaking you may need to feel that a person cares so much about you that your sex problems won't matter; that giving you the necessary time for lovemaking is not only not a bore but a positive joy; that it is the human being who really counts, not just the sex act he or she takes part in.

CASE STUDY *Kathryn & Martin*

Kathryn and Martin were both experienced lovers. Each of them knew exactly what they were doing when it came to lovemaking, but over the years Martin had grown so used to making love in a certain way that he found it difficult to climax when he made love with Kathryn.

Name:	KATHRYN
Age:	31
Marital status:	SINGLE
Occupation:	TEACHER

Kathryn was a 31-year-old teacher who had fallen in love with an older colleague after having had several lovers, including one long-term relationship of six years. She regarded herself as sexually experienced and felt surprised that she didn't know how to deal with the situation she found herself in.

"Martin is a very special man," she said. "He makes me feel beautiful, dynamic and sexy, but we have a problem in bed. Everything's fine for me. He's a fabulous, imaginative lover, knows exactly what to do and brings me to orgasm in just about any and every way imaginable. The trouble is, he only manages to climax with the greatest difficulty, and we can spend hours having intercourse before he can come. By the time we finish, I'm tired, sore, and — dare I say it — bored? Is there any way I could speed him up?"

Name:	MARTIN
Age:	50
Marital status:	SEPARATED
Occupation:	TEACHER

Martin had thick gray hair and an attractive, tanned face, but an air of fatigue. He had recently separated from his wife and revealed that there had been little sex in his marriage for many years. Kathryn was the first woman he had made love to, other than his wife, in twenty years.

"I didn't have a very active sex life during my marriage, but when we did get together I had no trouble at all in coming. Now, though, it's as if the sensation in my penis is blunted. When we start off I do feel very aroused, but turning her on takes time, and by the time she has climaxed my first impetus seems to have vanished. Of course, I've been used to lovemaking in a certain pattern with my wife, and I suppose not doing this is impeding me.

"Did my wife do anything differently from Kathryn? Well, yes, of course she did. One of the things I miss is that she used her hands on me a lot. For instance, she was quite rough with my penis."

THERAPIST'S ASSESSMENT

Both Kathryn and Martin were saying, independently of each other, that they wished the other would speed up a bit. Unfortunately for Kathryn, Martin was experiencing a period of readjustment after the end of his marriage, and he was finding it difficult to adjust to new lovemaking routines. Moreover, he, like many other older men, had difficulties with stimulation: it is perfectly common for men to need more stimulation as they grow older.

EXTRA STIMULATION
The extra stimulation that an older man often needs may take the form of additional visual stimulation, such as the use of blue movies or books, or it may involve physical stimulation such as very firm or vigorous handling of his genitals. Many a man likes attention paid to his penis and genitals by his partner's hand during intercourse, while others also need some anal and prostate gland stimulation in order to climax.

MUTUAL TRUST
Then, too, Martin and Kathryn may not have learned to trust one another sufficiently. Martin hadn't liked to suggest that he should go ahead and climax first during lovemaking, instead of taking time to stimulate Kathryn, because he felt it would prevent him from satisfying her. It hadn't occurred to him that Kathryn might not mind this, or that she might love him enough to tolerate a lack of satisfaction occasionally. Another thing that didn't occur to him was that even if he no longer had an erection, there are many enjoyable ways of satisfying a partner other than by intercourse.

SPEEDIER RESPONSE
Once all these new scenarios had been explored in counseling, Martin did allow more feeling to seep through into his consciousness and ultimately his penis. He managed to be upfront about the methods he preferred: like many men, he favored very rough handling of his penis, and once Kathryn understood this his response speeded up remarkably.

USING A VIBRATOR
Martin welcomed the suggestion of occasionally using a vibrator to give Kathryn an especially intense arousal. He liked the option this gave him, namely that if, on these occasions, she climaxed quickly, he could remain spontaneous with his early excitement.

My program for
INCREASING YOUR OPTIONS

Most of us enter into sexual relationships with little thought about what we want from them. One result is that often we don't end up doing what we want, nor do we get the sort of lover we really desire. Part of increasing your options is to know yourself, your own responses and those of your partner. And by slowly becoming more daring, either on your own or with a partner, you will gain more confidence, will become more assertive, will learn to cope with rejection better, and will go on to initiate sexual acts that you may have wanted to do but didn't have the confidence to suggest.

Stage 1 · LEARN MORE ABOUT EACH OTHER

Deliberately exploring yourself and your partner is the first step in learning what sexual options may exist for you. Self-pleasuring that leads to self-knowledge is vital, as is learning your partner's erogenous zones. Only by widening your knowledge of yourself and your partner can you give yourself choices.

EROGENOUS ZONES When you explore your partner's erogenous zones, start with the obvious ones such as nipples and genitals, and try out different ways of stimulating them. Then ask your partner about other, more subtle erogenous zones, and find out how he or she likes them to be stimulated.

After you have explored the erogenous zones that your partner is aware of, look for others: most people have more erogenous zones than they ever imagined.

Explore and learn about each other's erogenous zones. This will help you develop intimacy and mutual trust, creating a sound basis on which to build a more adventurous sex life

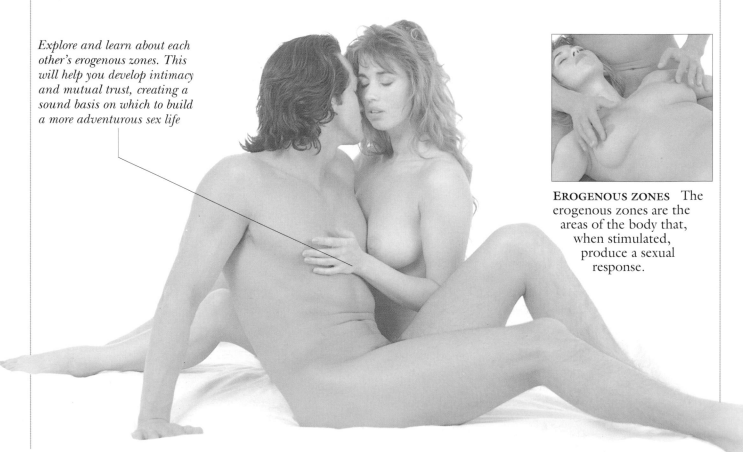

EROGENOUS ZONES The erogenous zones are the areas of the body that, when stimulated, produce a sexual response.

Stage 2 DISCOVER YOUR OPTIONS

There are a number of activities you can begin to experiment with to increase your sensuality and explore possibilities that may not have occurred to you before.

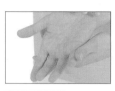

Sensual touch p28

STROKING Touching and stroking yourself and your partner are among the more obvious sources of sensual pleasure. Touch yourself slowly and sensuously after a hot bath, using sweet-smelling body lotions or oils and discovering your hidden erogenous zones. Stroke your partner from time to time, and in addition give "mental stroking" by regularly telling your partner, "I love you" and complementing him or her. Explain to your partner that you too would like to be touched and stroked, and share your feelings about this openly and freely.

MASTURBATION Learn to masturbate freely and with no guilt, and have sex only when you want to, not when you don't. Be choosy and seek the sort of sex experience that you desire, and don't be afraid to indulge in fantasy. Try expanding on your existing fantasies and bring in new ideas; if possible, find a fantasy that you can act out with your partner, remembering that you may have to adapt it slightly in order to cater to your partner's sexual preferences.

Be frank with your partner about what you would like to do, but be willing to drop the idea if your partner isn't enthusiastic about it, and consider any ideas and suggestions that your partner may have.

SEX WITHOUT INTERCOURSE Don't forget that there are plenty of non-intercourse sexual activities that you and your partner can share. These range from simply looking at and admiring each other's naked bodies to mutual masturbation and oral sex.

You can, of course, combine any or even all of these activities with intercourse. You might want to do this simply for the pleasure of it, or perhaps as a means of introducing an element of variety into your lovemaking so that you don't slip into a predictable routine that will inevitably become boring.

Either way, you will find that the sharing of non-intercourse sexual activities will add a new dimension of sensuality and intimacy to your relationship.

Stage 3 ADD MORE OPTIONS

Even when you and your partner have learned to discover your options, there is still room for expanding what the two of you have found possible to do in bed so far. Taking what you have already discovered as your starting point, you will find it easy to build up a wide variety of loving sexual practices.

INCREASE EROTICISM Every day, tell your lover what you love about him or her, and also tell yourself what it is you love about you. Add to the eroticism of your lovemaking by putting mirrors alongside your bed, so that you and your partner can watch yourselves making love. An extension of this idea is to record the sounds of your lovemaking on tape, or even to set up a camcorder or a home movie camera and recorder and make a movie of it.

SHARE SENSUAL EXPERIENCES Masturbate in front of your lover, and try a new sex position every few weeks. When you have time, take a shower or bath together, then massage each other with scented oils and give each other a foot massage. Other shared sensual experiences you might like to try include brushing and washing each other's hair, eating dinner together in the nude, fingerpainting each other's bodies, reading erotica together or out loud to each other, and sharing a vibrator.

MENTAL EROTICISM Eroticism is, of course, a mental as well as a physical phenomenon, and there are plenty of ways in which you and your partner can show your love for and attraction to each other without physical contact. For instance, you could send each other love letters or leave love notes in unexpected places, or describe sexual fantasies to each other in explicit detail. You could even arrange to meet in a bar or at some other suitable venue and pick each other up.

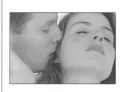

Fantasies pp138-143

SHEDDING INHIBITIONS Perhaps the main difficulty confronting people who are convinced that they are ineffective, and therefore couldn't carry out any of the suggestions mentioned above, is that of breaking away from their inhibitions. However, someone who is going through any experience of making overtures to a partner (or possible partner) is already making that essential breakthrough, even though they may not realize it.

SEXY UNDRESSING

Visual stimulation is extremely important to a man's arousal. A normal sex drive can be given an extra boost and a depressed one awakened by the sight of a female removing her clothes in a provocative way. A professional stripper will have had plenty of experience, and while no one expects you to be as good, you can improve your undressing technique enormously by regular practice in private in front of a full-length mirror.

Let a strap slip over your shoulder to hint at further disarray

Wear an underwire push-up bra to emphasize your breasts and cleavage

Rub your hand seductively up and down your thigh before removing your slip

Let some thigh show between the tops of your stockings and the bottom of your panties

SLIP OR CHEMISE Your order of undressing, once the outer layers have been removed, might focus on your slip. One that you can drop and step out of, while still wearing your high heels, is preferable to one that is pulled off over your head.

HIGH HEELS These are often a turn-on for men, because they make a woman's legs look longer and tend to push her buttocks to a sexier angle. (Try walking around the room in your underwear and heels, and see what effect it has on him.)

Keep hold of your slip as you step out of it, so that you can then throw it aside with the kind of dramatic gesture that a stripper would use

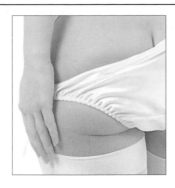

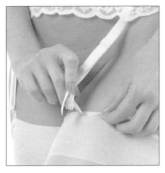

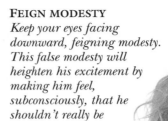

PANTIES   Pulling your panties off using only one hand looks more graceful than bending over and using both.

STOCKINGS AND GARTER BELT   Stockings and garter belts are always sexier than pantyhose, and high-cut briefs or tap pants, preferably silk ones, are sexier than ordinary cotton panties.

Teasingly thrust your leg forward so that your thigh obscures your genital area

STOCKING REMOVAL
Undoing garters allows you great opportunities for making delicious shapes with your legs, and slowly peeling the stocking away from a perfectly groomed limb is extremely erotic.

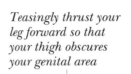

Adopt positions that you know are a turn-on

TAKING YOUR BRA OFF
Being reluctant to disclose your breasts, and teasing a little about whether you really are going to take your upper garment away or not before finally daring to do so, will be far more erotic than if you just suddenly whip it off.

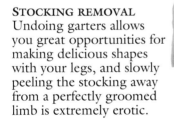

Use your fingers and hands to stroke your legs seductively as you slip your stockings off

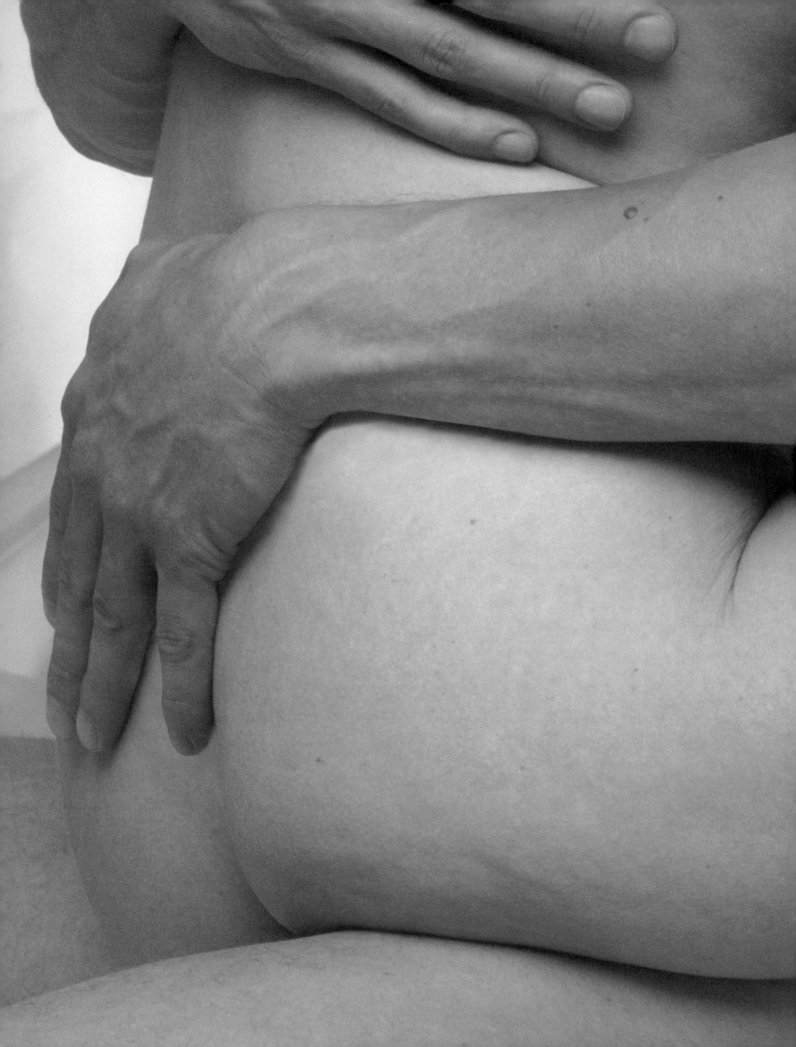

5
CHAPTER

A SEXUAL BANQUET

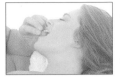

Eating and making love are two of life's great sensual activities. The mouth, one of the most versatile parts of the body, is capable of giving and experiencing pleasure in a variety of ways. To create a sexual banquet, the kissing, sucking on, nibbling, and gentle biting of a lover's body can be imaginatively combined with the erotic application of specially selected foods to create an experience that is tasty in every sense. This touch of the exotic should help to widen sexual horizons in a most enjoyable way.

TREAT YOUR PARTNER
As a special sensual surprise — say when your partner has just emerged from a relaxing bath — prepare a dish of fruits and other delicious fare, and serve with some chilled wine.

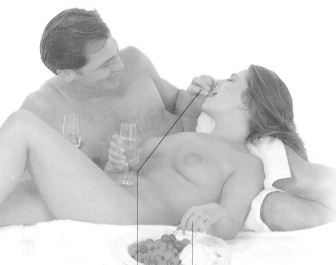

Make the experience more erotic by feeding your partner

Take turns offering food to each other

POUR ON THE PLEASURE
A little honey, syrup, or some champagne feels good going on over the breasts and navel.

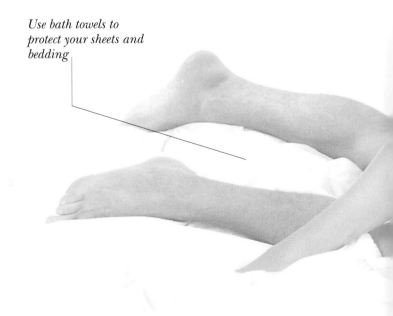

Use bath towels to protect your sheets and bedding

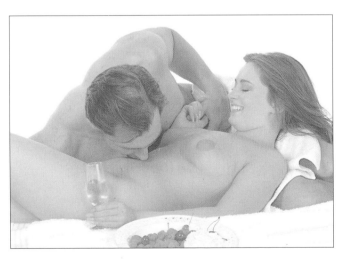

USE YOUR MOUTH CREATIVELY Lick and suck up the honey, syrup, or wine from your partner's body, making exaggerated gestures with your tongue. Long sweeps of your tongue's rough surface will feel incredibly sensuous and are bound to make your partner feel good.

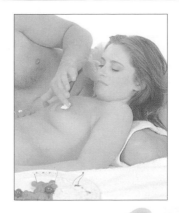

APPLY BODY "PAINT"
Cream can be dabbed onto your partner's nipples using slow circular movements, and can be sucked off afterward.

Let her know she looks good enough to eat

Move teasingly close to her genitals

STRATEGIC POSITIONING
Place some fruit close to your partner's genitals and eat it off him or her in a provocative way.

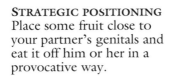

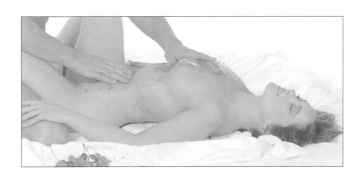

NO HOLDS BARRED Smear your partner all over with soft fruit, crushing it against his or her naked body and rubbing it slowly and sensuously up and down and around in circles (see left). You can even heighten the feelings of erotic intimacy by feeding each other mouth-to-mouth while continuing to caress each other through the fruit. When you are both thoroughly aroused and ready, bring your sexual banquet to a glorious climax by making love while continuing to massage each other with the crushed fruit (below).

Seductively press the fruit against your partner's body

Let your partner see how much you are enjoying this novel experience

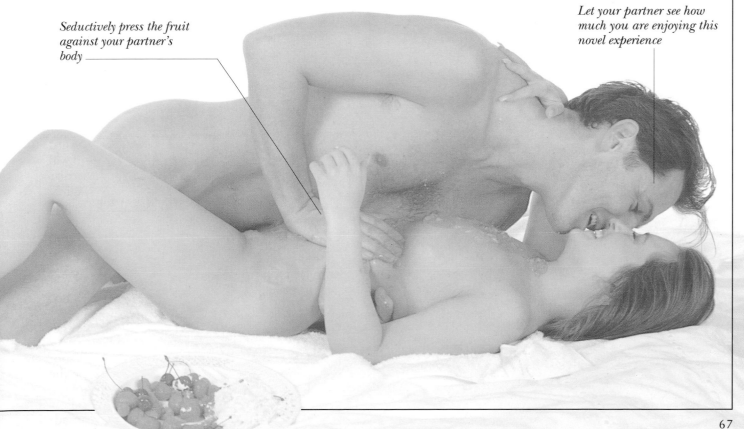

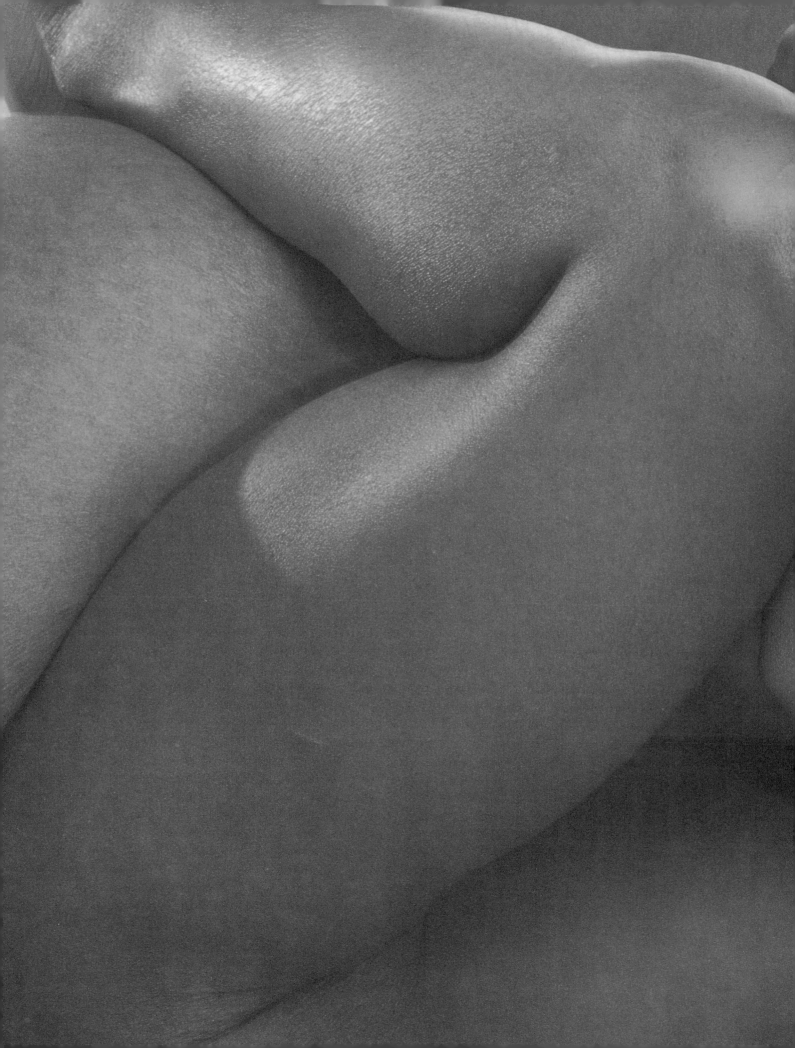

CHAPTER

6

HOW CAN I ASK FOR WHAT I WANT IN BED?

"How can the more timid reach the level of self-confidence that allows us to ask for exactly what we want? The secret is to start in small ways, tackling easier tasks first and harder ones later once our confidence has begun to rise."

ONE OF THE common sources of problems within relationships is a lack of communication between the two partners, and this failure to communicate is especially rife when it comes to sexual matters. Many women have unsatisfactory sex lives because they cannot bring themselves to discuss with their partners the subject of what they need in bed.

In an ideal world, men would recognize and be sensitive to the sexual needs of their partners and would do their best to ensure that these needs were met. But men are often unaware that their partners are not getting true sexual fulfillment. They don't notice it, and their partners are too shy, or for some reason reluctant, to raise the subject.

The best way to overcome these difficulties in a relationship is for the woman to take the initiative and learn how to express her needs clearly but tactfully, and to explain to her man what her needs are and what he can do to meet them.

The first step is for her to become more assertive. She must learn how to feel comfortable discussing the subject. Once she is able to talk freely to her partner about sex, she will find it easier to take a more active role in their lovemaking, and that will increase the pleasure for both of them.

CASE STUDY *Irene & Tom*

Tom was a hurried lover and never quite got Irene to orgasm. She was fairly certain that if only he would continue stimulating her with his fingers for a little longer she could come. But once he had reached his orgasm she never liked to ask him, and the result of this was that he never knew that she was physically capable of climax — so he didn't learn how to get her there.

Name:	IRENE
Age:	22
Marital status:	SINGLE
Occupation:	RECEPTIONIST

Irene, who was in her second sexual relationship, felt strongly that she wasn't getting as much physical pleasure out of her love affair as she would have liked.

"I've never had an orgasm," she said. "But I've read enough about it to know I'm missing something. Tom's a great guy, but he's always in a hurry. Not just with sex, but with his whole life. He's a salesman, and very ambitious – he's off to work early, and he telephones people half the evenings we spend together, which since we don't even live together is a bit much. I've hardly started in bed before he's all done. I think I could have a climax with him if only he'd slow down a little, but I find it terribly hard to ask for any changes. I'm scared he'll think it'll mean he's no good in bed, and then he'll reject me. It's not that. I need a different pace. But I can't face asking for it."

Name:	TOM
Age:	26
Marital status:	SINGLE
Occupation:	SALESMAN

Tom was dressed in a business suit and carrying both a briefcase and a sample case. On several occasions he glanced at his watch. "I'm here because Irene asked me to come. She seems to have quite a sex problem, which obviously I'd like to help her with. Naturally I'd prefer her to have orgasms with me, but to be quite fair she's always seemed to enjoy sex anyway. Yes, I'm pretty serious about her. I wouldn't be here if I wasn't. We're intending to get engaged in four months' time. Two of her brothers are good friends of mine, and I think a lot of her family.

"I've had several girlfriends before, none of whom had this difficulty. But I never felt serious about any of them. Irene may be quiet, but she's an extremely bright girl. I find her really interesting to talk to, and I get good feelings from being with her. Yes, I want to do well. I'm trying to make as many sales now as possible in order to get enough money to serve as a deposit on a house. I want my wife and kids to have as high a standard of living as possible."

THERAPIST'S ASSESSMENT

There were two issues to deal with here. One was that Irene needed to learn how to ask difficult questions when she feared the outcome. The second was that, from the sound of it, Tom was not only not paying enough attention to Irene's needs, he was also rushing his climax.

LEARNING TO SLOW DOWN

Tom's hurry with life in general, with his career, with sex, and with answering questions on Irene's behalf in particular, was pointed out. Perhaps because his hurry had already been touched on in the session, he quickly grasped the point — he needed to give Irene more space to be herself. In answering for Irene he had, he felt, been protecting her.

It was pointed out that the person he was really protecting, when doing this, was his childhood self. Since the original family set-up no longer existed, except in his own head, this was no longer necessary. Tom visibly relaxed as this was recognized and Irene voiced her sympathy for him with warmth.

Tom swore to turn over a new leaf and a private code word was worked out between the couple for Irene to say, should Tom fall into his old habits. In addition, Tom agreed to try to prolong his orgasm, if necessary using sex therapy methods such as the squeeze (see page 59) in order to do so.

BECOMING HEALTHILY SELFISH

Irene's first task was to learn how to have orgasms through self-stimulation (see page 232). Once she had discovered what her sexual response consisted of, she was then in a much better position to take this information into the relationship and share it with Tom. The second was to learn the basic principles of assertion training by using simple exercises that helped her to ask for what she wanted, even in situations she found difficult, and to apply these when in bed with her partner.

Tom still needed a bit of restraining through the following months, but he learned to slow himself down enough to give Irene opportunity to start being herself, instead of a shadow of him. He also learned to enjoy stimulating her and discovered that this could be highly arousing for himself. The sex improved enormously, as did the general level of communication between them, and in a few months' time it was a much happier couple who announced their engagement without apprehension.

My program for
SEXUAL ASSERTIVENESS

Assertiveness helps us deal with tricky situations. It establishes feelings of self-value and importance, and assures us that it's all right to change our minds and normal to make mistakes. Becoming sexually assertive means coping with situations that are uncomfortable to you, knowing what you are allowed to have or do, and finally putting your assertiveness into action.

Stage 1 — DEALING WITH WHAT MAKES YOU UNEASY

The first thing to do is to clarify in your own mind what your problem situations are. Make a list of the situations (they don't all have to be sexual ones) with which you find it hard to cope. Then shuffle the list into an order of priority with the most difficult situations at the top and the least difficult at the bottom. Starting at the bottom, practice acting through each situation with a friend. If, because it is intimate, there is a particular situation you do not want to rehearse with someone else, practice alone in front of your mirror and tape record your voice to make sure you express yourself clearly and convincingly.

When you have gained confidence in this way, you will be ready to cope with the real thing. Take a deep breath and try to deal with it in the way that you handled it when you were practicing, bearing in mind the "assertiveness bill of rights."

Stage 2 — SAYING DIRTY WORDS OUT LOUD

There is a famous training technique, used to get professional counselors comfortable with talking about sex, that consists of showing a blitz of films about sexuality, which are then discussed. One of the first movies is of an actor simply reading through a list; the list goes on and on. Any film of a man reading a list would be bizarre, but this one is particularly so because the list consists of dirty words.

Your first reaction at the start of the movie is incredulity and shock, but what happens as you hear so much foul language formally presented is that in the end, as you sit there and listen, none of it affects you anymore.

You've simply gotten used to the experience. The process of being exposed to something for so long that it no longer affects you is called desensitization.

DIRTY WORDS Dirty words carry with them negative connotations — a sort of negative charge. If you should hear one or more of these words you may well immediately think with condemnation of the object described. But the fact is that these so-called "dirty" words are almost invariably words that describe

THE ASSERTIVENESS BILL OF RIGHTS

• I have the right to judge my own behavior, thoughts, and emotions, and to take responsibility for their initiation and consequences.

• I have the right to offer no reasons or excuses to justify my behavior.

• I have the right to decide whether or not I am, or should be, responsible for finding a solution to other people's problems.

• I have the right to change my mind.

• I have the right to make mistakes and be responsible for them.

• I have the right to say, "I don't know."

• I have the right to be independent of the goodwill of other people while I am dealing with a tricky situation or problem.

• I have the right to be illogical in making decisions.

• I have the right to say, "I don't understand" and to ask for information.

genitalia and sexual activity. Small wonder, perhaps, that we tend to look upon sex as a negative experience to be kept very private. The harm in that is that if we are inhibited, we remain that way because we never dare talk about the problems.

TALKING EXPLICITLY   The logic behind desensitization is that it reduces the negative charge of the words to a point where we can think objectively about the subject described by them. It is obviously desirable to be able to talk about sex without negative feelings.

If you find it hard to talk explicitly about sex without extreme self-consciousness, that might inhibit you from talking frankly about what you want in bed. To make it easier for you to talk freely about sex, draw up a check-list of "loaded" words and practice saying them out loud in front of a mirror. When you can say them without cringing you are going to find it a whole lot easier to discuss sex.

Stage 3 DEMONSTRATING YOUR ASSERTIVENESS

A woman can demonstrate her assertiveness in many ways, including the way in which she undresses. For example, the body language of

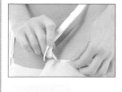

Sexy un-dressing p54

a good professional stripper will indicate self-love, and she will often fondle herself, with no apparent self-consciousness, as she looks over her shoulder at her audience. She will not use body language that cringes, or attempt to hide parts of herself. No one is suggesting, of course, that you should bump and grind, but gaining a clear idea of a smooth way in which to disrobe, and of the body language that will make this most provocative to your partner, can't hurt.

It is definitely more erotic to be undressed by someone than to do it yourself, and undressing your partner demonstrates your

assertiveness as well as being very stimulating for him. If you are going to be effective at disrobing your partner, you need first to have had practice in undoing things and second to know the right order in which to undo them. For example, your man won't thank you if you get his trousers and briefs off first and then leave him exposed while you work on the upper half.

TAKING THE LEAD   Another sign of assertiveness is taking the lead during sex. Many men don't expect their women to want to do anything other than be passive. It can be a surprise when she turns to him after they have made love and says, "That was lovely. Now I want to make love to you." However, many men are so conditioned to be active that they find it almost impossible to lie back and accept pleasure. To overcome this, turn the lovemaking session into a sort of sensual massage. It is also worth being assertive if your partner climaxes before you, leaving you unfulfilled. If you are confident in bed you could, at a discreet interval after his climax, say simply, "Would you rub my clitoris again like you were doing before? It felt wonderful and I'd like a climax now." The result would be that he would then learn something important about satisfying you sexually, and you would feel good both for asking for pleasure and for receiving it.

Taking the lead p74

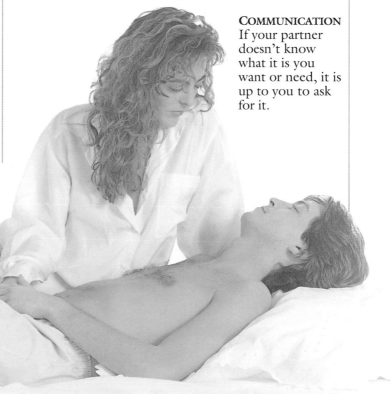

COMMUNICATION If your partner doesn't know what it is you want or need, it is up to you to ask for it.

TAKING THE LEAD IN LOVEMAKING

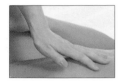 *Many men don't expect their women to want to do anything other than be passive, and they are so conditioned to be active that they find it almost impossible to lie back and accept pleasure. The best way of overcoming this is to confront it openly and turn the session into a version of "Me, Jane; you, Tarzan."*

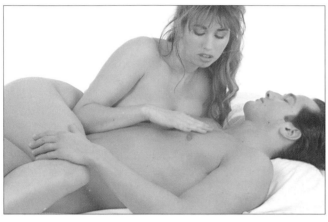

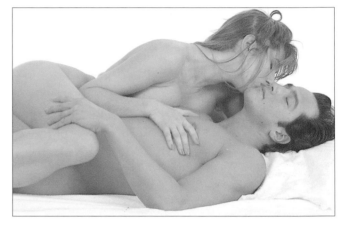

1 MAKE THE FIRST MOVE Slide playfully on top of your man, stroking him erotically and rubbing your body sensually against his.

2 START TO AROUSE HIM Before he gets a chance to heave you off him, move sensuously down his naked body, kissing and stroking his torso.

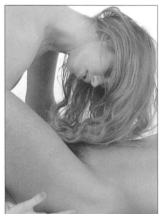

3 TICKLE HIM If you have longish hair you can sweep across his genitals with it, dragging your mane across his abdomen and down over his penis.

Press the length of your body against his so that he feels surrounded by you

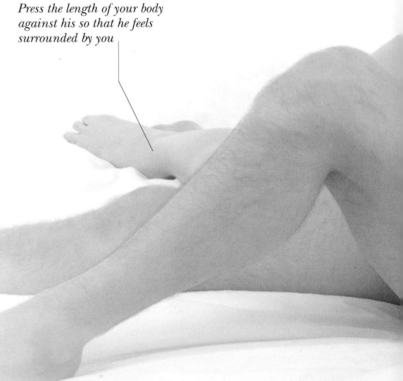

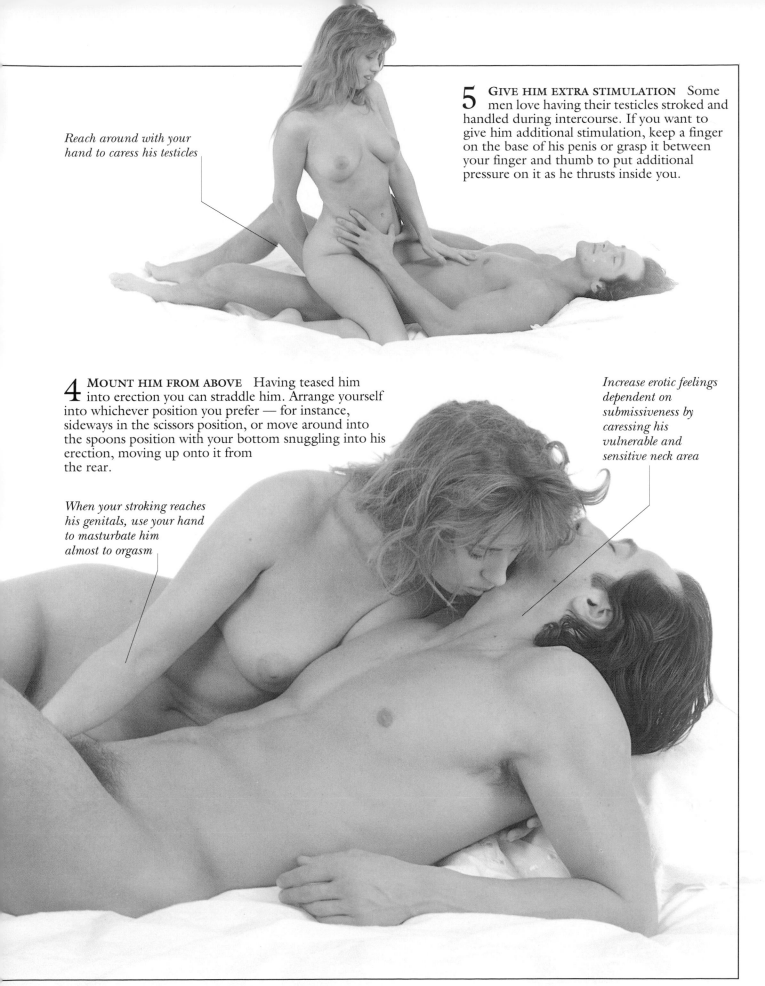

Reach around with your hand to caress his testicles

5 **GIVE HIM EXTRA STIMULATION** Some men love having their testicles stroked and handled during intercourse. If you want to give him additional stimulation, keep a finger on the base of his penis or grasp it between your finger and thumb to put additional pressure on it as he thrusts inside you.

4 **MOUNT HIM FROM ABOVE** Having teased him into erection you can straddle him. Arrange yourself into whichever position you prefer — for instance, sideways in the scissors position, or move around into the spoons position with your bottom snuggling into his erection, moving up onto it from the rear.

When your stroking reaches his genitals, use your hand to masturbate him almost to orgasm

Increase erotic feelings dependent on submissiveness by caressing his vulnerable and sensitive neck area

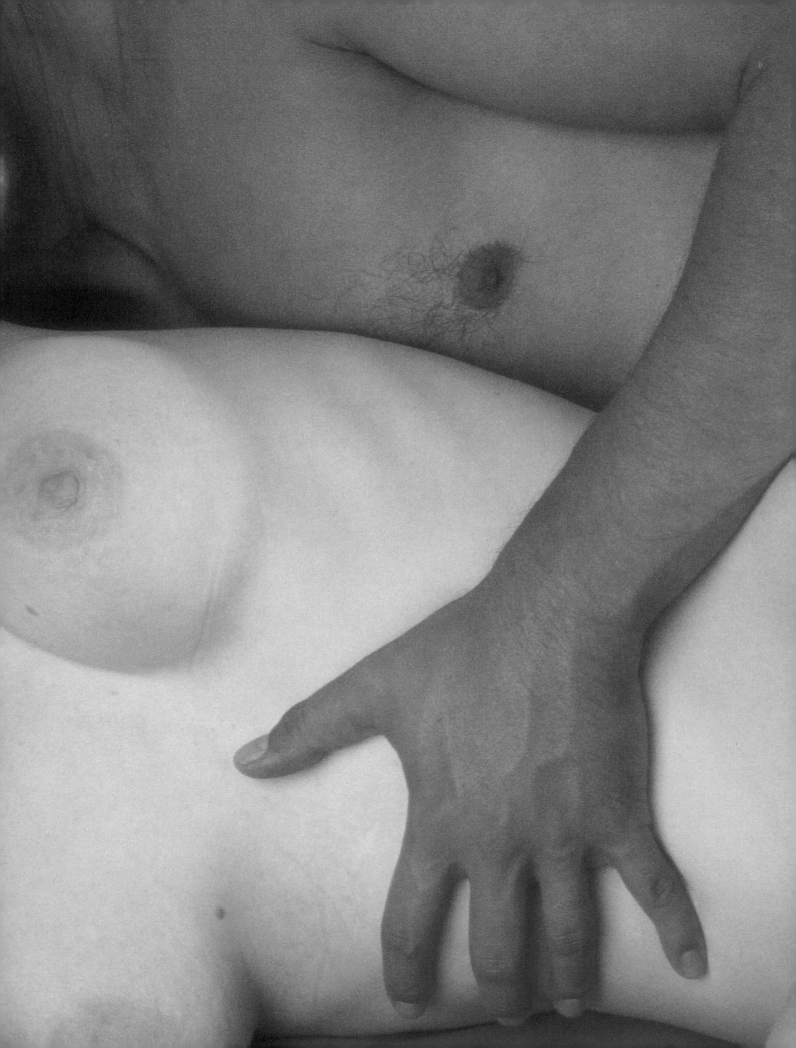

CHAPTER

7

HOW CAN I MAKE LOVE~ MAKING MORE INTIMATE?

"Opening your innermost self to your partner can be difficult, but it is essential if you want your relationship to flourish and grow."

JUST BECAUSE two people make love does not, surprisingly enough, guarantee that they are intimate. Intimacy is a quality that grows through a sharing of feelings; it heightens all aspects of the relationship and is the main ingredient responsible for turning sex into an ecstatic experience as opposed to a pleasurable but uninspiring one.

In order to achieve intimacy we need to be brave enough to reveal our innermost selves to our partners, which is something that many people find difficult to do.

This difficulty may arise for many people because they worry that their inner selves might be unacceptable, or because they feel that revealing too much about themselves to another person (even though that person may be someone who is very close to them) will make them vulnerable in some way.

Creating the conditions in which your lover feels safe enough to talk about deep, inner feelings helps him or her to overcome such fears, and so does the ability to open up and share your own feelings.

CASE STUDY *Maria & Jack*

Although Maria and Jack had known each other only a short time, they got along very well together, both in bed and out of it. But they found it difficult to be truly intimate with each other and to confide their innermost thoughts and feelings, and that left them both dissatisfied.

Name:	MARIA
Age:	28
Marital status:	SINGLE
Occupation:	HAIRDRESSER

Maria was from an Italian-American family, and her brother, two sisters, and most of her cousins were already married. She had some strongly independent ideas about life, though, and owned her own car and house.

"I don't have any difficulty in attracting men," she said, "I'm dating an extremely interesting guy at the moment. He's ambitious and bright and I'm learning a lot from him. He'd be a suitable husband but, as happened with the last couple of boyfriends I had, I can't really be myself with him when we go to bed.

"It's not that I'm afraid of talking about sex or of making sexual suggestions, but there is a feeling, at the end of lovemaking, that things aren't quite right. I don't feel really relaxed, even though I've climaxed. Afterward, I feel a million miles away from him. I look at him and wonder what he's thinking. And because he never opens up to me, I don't really reveal my inner self to him. I'd like to. But I'm not quite sure how to."

Name:	JACK
Age:	37
Marital status:	SINGLE
Occupation:	TRANSPORT MANAGER

Jack was brisk and confident, excellent at managing staff and working for one of the most efficient companies in his field. His career record was excellent, but his record with girlfriends was not so good. There had been several live-in partners in the past, and Jack was unsure about why these affairs had not lasted.

"I do like Maria a great deal," he told me. "And I know what she's talking about. I'd love to feel really relaxed with someone too, but it's not easy for me. I seriously want to marry and have children, but I don't believe in divorce. My parents got divorced when I was twelve, and my mother was devastated by it.

"For me, living with someone is one thing, but marriage is for life. And since that's the case, it's really got to work out, right from the start."

THERAPIST'S ASSESSMENT

Both Maria and Jack were complaining about a lack of intimacy. Sex for them was pleasant, but each of them felt that it would have to provide them with something more than simple physical satisfaction if their partnership was going to be other than temporary.

Their anxieties were brought to a head by the needs of each of them to make a permanent relationship. But since both were highly assertive and capable, their sense of helplessness was accentuated because this was one of the few situations in their lives where neither of them had a clue how to proceed.

FOSTERING INTIMACY

Intimacy is fostered both by the romance of the surroundings and by the ability of those involved to be open and self-disclosing. Because Maria and Jack were busy, capable individuals, they had learned to compartmentalize their lives. This worked excellently as a method of getting efficiently through their workloads, but it also meant that they were poor at sharing their feelings and their experiences with each other.

Since Maria and Jack were both also highly competitive they had learned, early on, not to reveal anything that might make them vulnerable, for fear that it would be used against them. During my individual discussions with them, I learned that there were, in fact, many things about both of them that, if they were revealed, would make them feel vulnerable.

SELF-DISCLOSURE

In order to open themselves to each other, reaching to their vulnerable inner selves, the couple needed to learn how to self-disclose. I warned them that it was going to feel extremely risky trying to do this, since it meant exposing soft parts of the ego, and that if they were going to succeed, each would have to give a great deal of reassurance to the other.

REASSURANCE

Maria and Jack learned how to give reassurance to each other by using comforting, loving words and touch, and how to get each other to self-disclose and express deeply personal thoughts and emotions. Maria and Jack followed through with these suggestions and ended up with a deeper and more tender relationship, a good basis for marriage.

My program for
INCREASING THE PHYSICAL
SIDE OF INTIMACY

On the previous pages I've suggested methods of reassuring and opening up to each other in the sharing of feelings. On these pages I suggest you play doctors, using a therapy sequence called the Sexological Exam, which I first learned about in the United States. This helps couples bring their genital sensuality into focus and, in the course of doing so, produces a sometimes extraordinary experience of discovery that draws them closer together. If you need an excuse, to help you to get started, pretend it's a game — you are the doctor, he is your patient, and he lies on a bed in a warm room while you examine him.

Stage 1   BREASTS AND NIPPLES

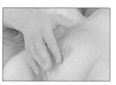

Sexological Exam p82

In the Sexological Exam, either partner can examine the other: on these two pages we show how she can examine him. Begin by finding out how his breasts and nipples respond to touching and stroking. Gently stroke each breast, then stroke or lightly press around the area of each nipple, using your fingertips. If his nipples become firm and erect, that shows that they are sensitive to stimulation. And if small pale spots appear on his erect nipples, this indicates high arousal.

Stage 2   PUBIC HAIR PATTERN

After examining your partner's breasts and nipples, transfer your attention to his pubic hair. Examine the hair's abundance and texture, and the area that it covers. Pubic hair patterns and thicknesses vary greatly from one man to another, taking a variety of shapes ranging from a sparse amount of hair just above the penis to a luxuriant growth stretching from the abdomen down to the genitals and onto the upper leg.

Pubic hair growth is commonly associated with the amount of free-ranging testosterone (a sex hormone) circulating in the body, and large amounts of testosterone may result in an abundance of body and pubic hair, at the same time causing baldness on the head.

Stage 3   THE PENIS

Hold your partner's penis in one hand and ask him to point out the areas that are most sensitive. Note where these are and ask what stimulation works best for him in these areas. Let him show you, then repeat the stimulation yourself. Please note, however, that the intention is not to bring him to orgasm, but to clarify for both of you his penile sensitivity.

PENIS SHAPE   Note the shape of his penis. Contrary to what many people believe, the appearance of a man's penis is as individual as the appearance of his face: penises don't all look the same. Ask him on which side he prefers to wear his penis when dressed, and ask if one side feels more sensitive than the other.

THE FORESKIN   If he is uncircumcised, ask him to show you how far back he can comfortably move his foreskin. If he is circumcised, look carefully at the exposed penis where the foreskin would have been and check this for scarring. If there is scarring, ask him what kind of sensation he feels in this area.

THE URETHRA   Look at the head of the penis. The urethra, the tiny slit from which your partner urinates and ejaculates, should be a healthy red color. On the underside of the penis, at the head, is a central ridge of skin called the frenulum. See if this is unbroken or if it is broken or scarred, and ask your partner what kind of sensation he experiences here.

THE PERINEUM Ring the base of the penis with your fingers and ask your partner what specific sensation there is here, if any. Trace your fingers lightly down his testicles and underneath them, where you will encounter the perineum. The perineum is the area between the testicles and the anus (on a woman, the perineum is the area between the vagina and anus), and it is often rich in nerve endings and so may be very sensitive to being touched or stroked. Gently run your fingers along the ridge of the perineum, and ask him how it feels to be stroked there.

Stage 4 THE ANUS

Imagine his anus to be a clock and press gently but firmly at the hour positions around it. Ask him if any of the areas feel sensitive: if they do, remember them when stimulating your partner during later lovemaking.

Finally, ask your partner to help you practise the squeeze technique on him (page 59), so that both of you can learn thorough control over his erection and ejaculation.

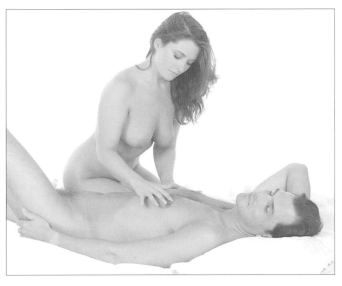

ANAL REGION Check the response of your partner's anal region by pressing gently but firmly at the hour positions around his anus. Imagine the point on the rim of his anus that is nearest his penis is at the 12 o'clock position. The most sensitive parts of his anus — those that produce the most sensation when they are pressed — will probably be the ten o'clock and two o'clock positions.

BREASTS AND NIPPLES The exam begins with a check on how your partner's breasts and nipples respond to stimulation. Stroke or lightly press around the area of the nipples to see if they become erect.

GENITAL STROKES Get your partner to show you where the most sensitive parts of his penis are and ask him to demonstrate to you how best to stimulate them, but remember that the object of the exercise is to gain information, not to bring him to orgasm.

Use a gentle touch when you are probing your partner's most sensitive parts

PRIVACY AND COMFORT
To do the Sexological Exam in comfort, you need privacy and a warm, draft-free room

Ask him for information and in return tell him what your own impressions are

THE SEXOLOGICAL EXAM

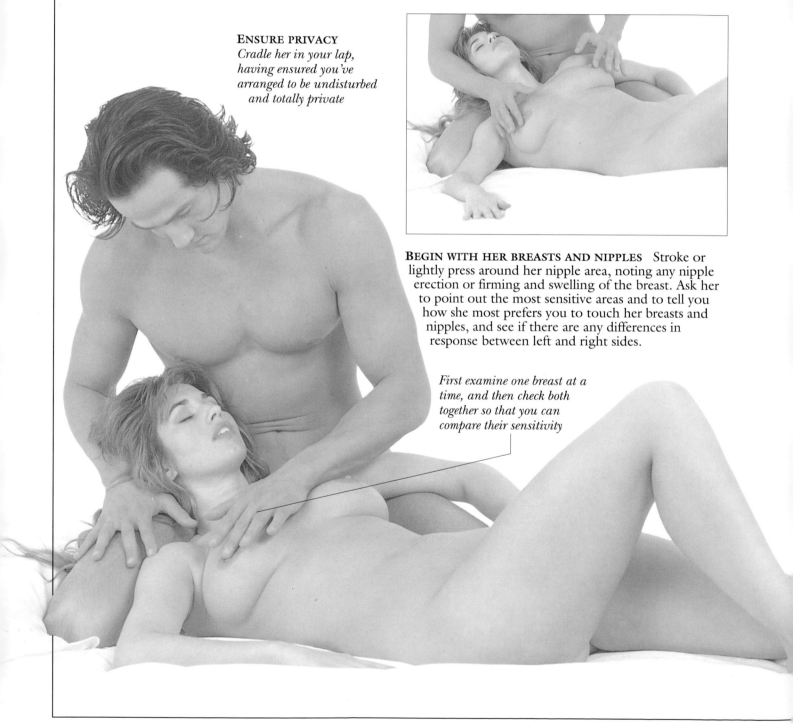

Exploring each other's "private parts" will bring you and your partner a new awareness of your genital sensuality, helping you to open up to each other and share your feelings more easily. You each in turn play the role of doctor, examining your partner's body to get to know it intimately, and asking questions about how your partner responds to being touched and caressed in his or her most sensitive areas. Here we show how a man can examine his partner; for how she can examine him, see pages 80-81.

ENSURE PRIVACY
Cradle her in your lap, having ensured you've arranged to be undisturbed and totally private

BEGIN WITH HER BREASTS AND NIPPLES Stroke or lightly press around her nipple area, noting any nipple erection or firming and swelling of the breast. Ask her to point out the most sensitive areas and to tell you how she most prefers you to touch her breasts and nipples, and see if there are any differences in response between left and right sides.

First examine one breast at a time, and then check both together so that you can compare their sensitivity

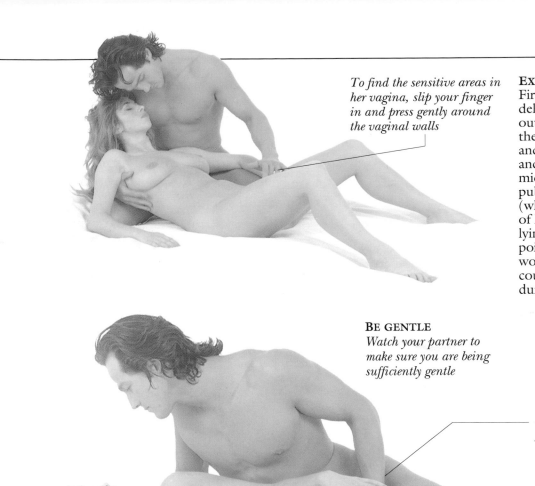

To find the sensitive areas in her vagina, slip your finger in and press gently around the vaginal walls

EXAMINE HER GENITALS
First place your fingers deliberately but gently on the outside of her labia, then at the opening of the vagina and just inside the vagina, and then on the base, the middle, and top of the pubococcygeus muscle (which is located on the floor of her vagina when she is lying on her back). At each point, ask her how much she would like it if your penis could hit that particular spot during intercourse.

BE GENTLE
Watch your partner to make sure you are being sufficiently gentle

Before you examine your partner's vagina and anus, lubricate your fingers with KY Jelly. Wash your hands immediately after exploring the anus

PROBE AROUND HER ANUS Imagine her anus to be a clock and press gently but firmly at the hour positions around it, asking her which feel the most sensitive: the ten o'clock and two o'clock positions are often the areas of greatest sexual stimulation (12 o'clock is the point closest to the vagina). The perineum, between the anus and vagina, is rich in nerve endings and so is always sensitive to stimulation.

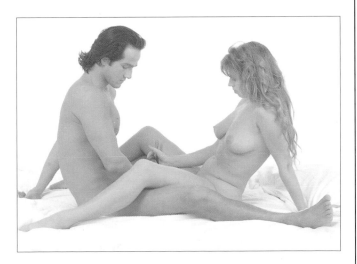

USING A MIRROR Give your partner a mirror so that she can see her genitals. Together, explore the outer and inner labia, and part them to reveal her clitoris and urethra and the entrance to her vagina.

83

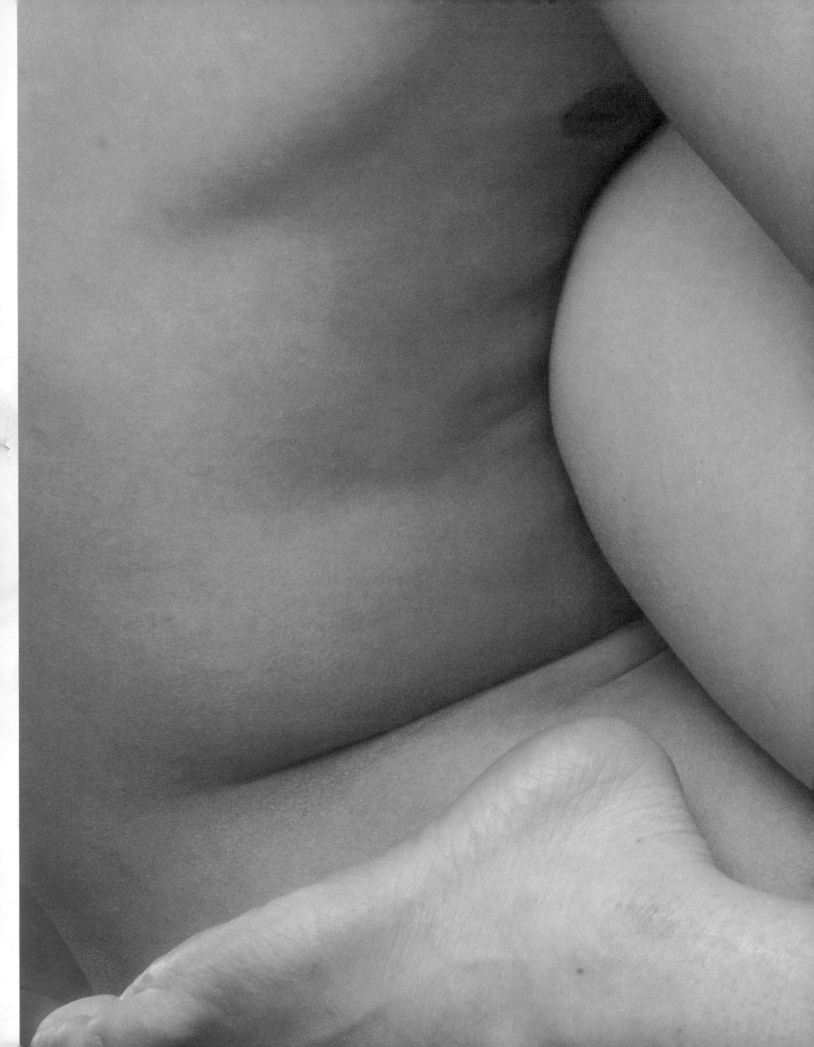

CHAPTER 8

MUTUAL MASTURBATION WITHOUT INTERCOURSE

Intercourse is not the only means to sexual excitement and satisfaction — skilled and loving mutual masturbation will also do the trick. Back in the days before contraception, young people went in for "heavy petting," which consisted of sex without intercourse. Most of the sexual stimulation was done by hand, and it took many sessions to get familiar with each other. This was a bonus because it meant there was time to develop trust and to build up knowledge of a partner's body and responses.

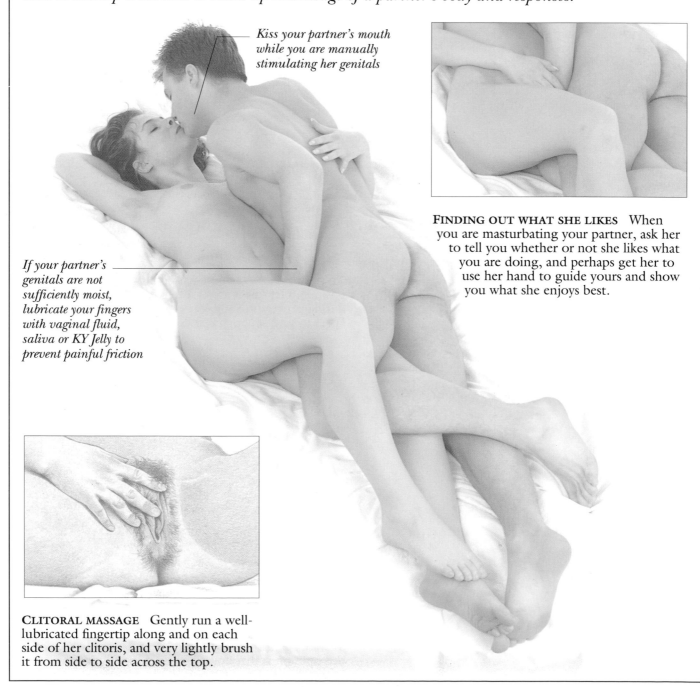

Kiss your partner's mouth while you are manually stimulating her genitals

If your partner's genitals are not sufficiently moist, lubricate your fingers with vaginal fluid, saliva or KY Jelly to prevent painful friction

FINDING OUT WHAT SHE LIKES When you are masturbating your partner, ask her to tell you whether or not she likes what you are doing, and perhaps get her to use her hand to guide yours and show you what she enjoys best.

CLITORAL MASSAGE Gently run a well-lubricated fingertip along and on each side of her clitoris, and very lightly brush it from side to side across the top.

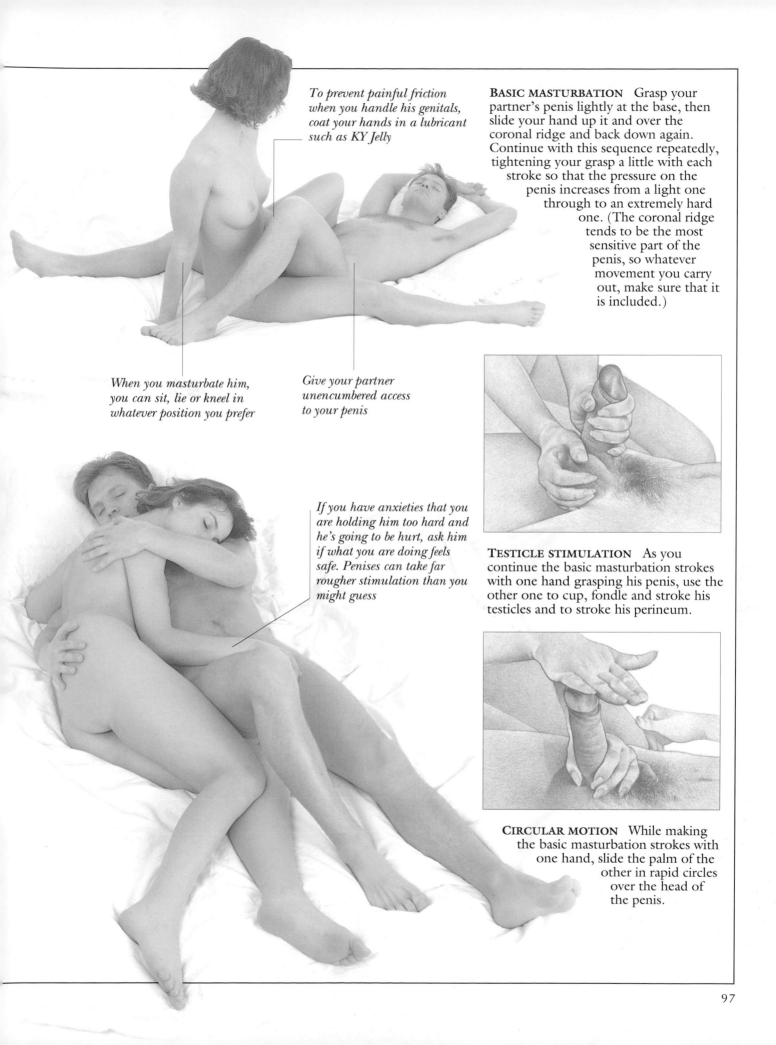

To prevent painful friction when you handle his genitals, coat your hands in a lubricant such as KY Jelly

BASIC MASTURBATION Grasp your partner's penis lightly at the base, then slide your hand up it and over the coronal ridge and back down again. Continue with this sequence repeatedly, tightening your grasp a little with each stroke so that the pressure on the penis increases from a light one through to an extremely hard one. (The coronal ridge tends to be the most sensitive part of the penis, so whatever movement you carry out, make sure that it is included.)

When you masturbate him, you can sit, lie or kneel in whatever position you prefer

Give your partner unencumbered access to your penis

If you have anxieties that you are holding him too hard and he's going to be hurt, ask him if what you are doing feels safe. Penises can take far rougher stimulation than you might guess

TESTICLE STIMULATION As you continue the basic masturbation strokes with one hand grasping his penis, use the other one to cup, fondle and stroke his testicles and to stroke his perineum.

CIRCULAR MOTION While making the basic masturbation strokes with one hand, slide the palm of the other in rapid circles over the head of the penis.

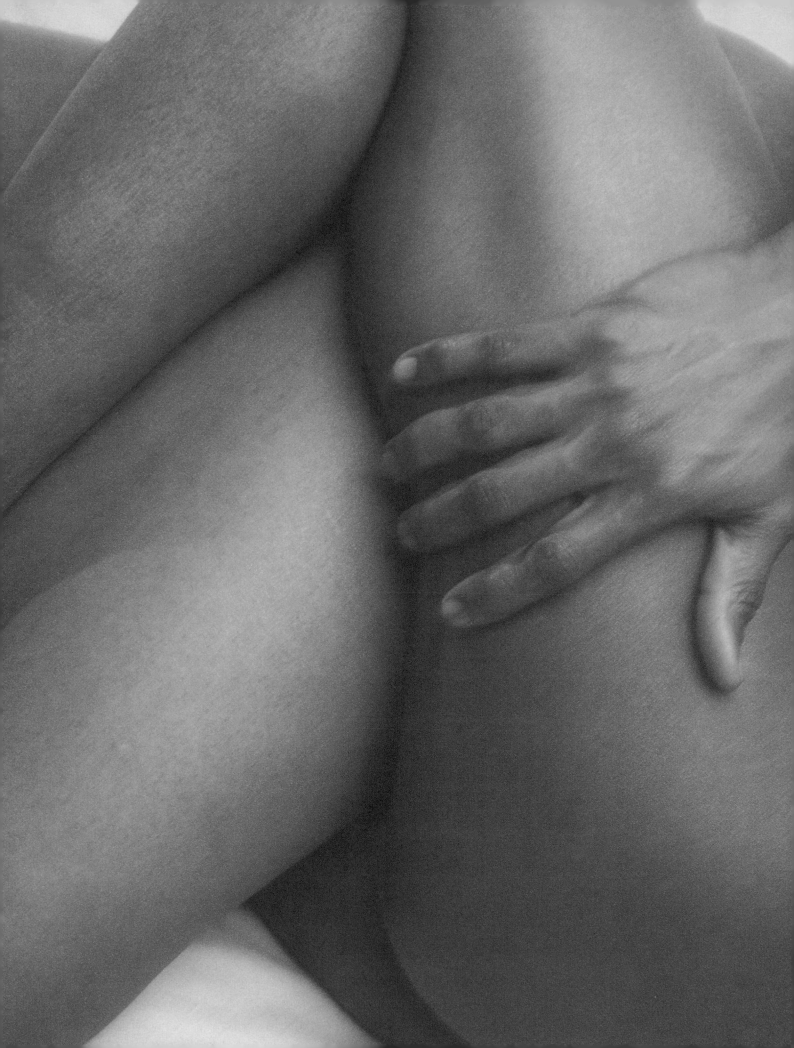

CHAPTER 9

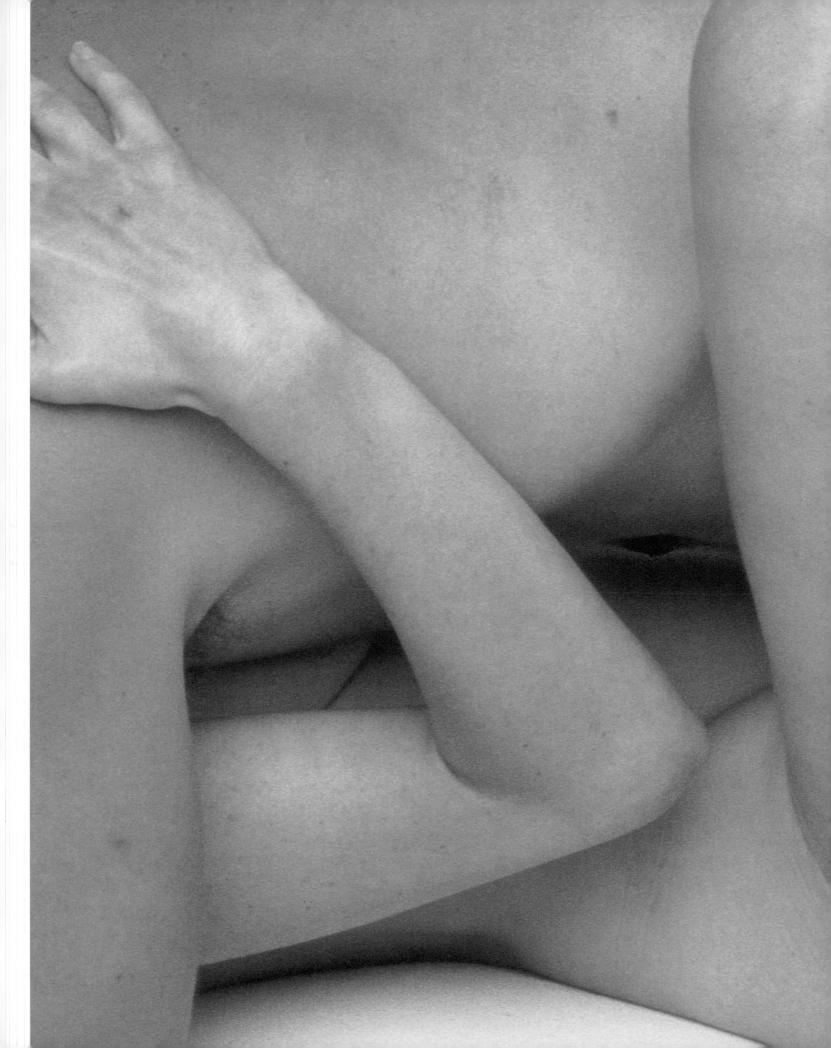

CHAPTER

10

BEYOND THE BEDROOM

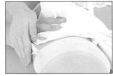

Most couples don't think twice about where they make love in the early stages of romance, but rigid patterns tend to set in. All too soon, lovemaking is restricted to the bedroom. Fortunately variety — necessary for the continued vigor of long-term relationships — can easily be reintroduced simply by changing the setting.

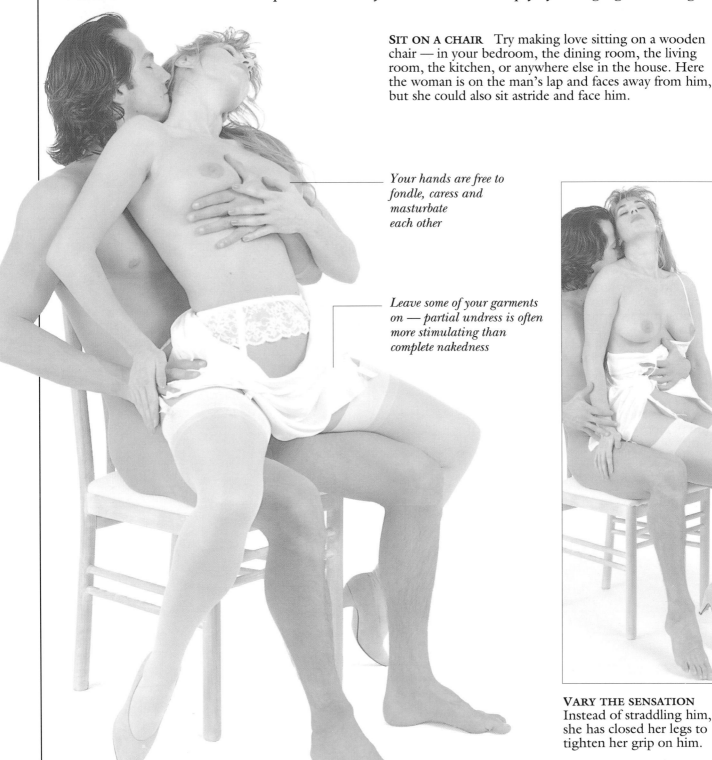

SIT ON A CHAIR Try making love sitting on a wooden chair — in your bedroom, the dining room, the living room, the kitchen, or anywhere else in the house. Here the woman is on the man's lap and faces away from him, but she could also sit astride and face him.

Your hands are free to fondle, caress and masturbate each other

Leave some of your garments on — partial undress is often more stimulating than complete nakedness

VARY THE SENSATION
Instead of straddling him, she has closed her legs to tighten her grip on him.

118

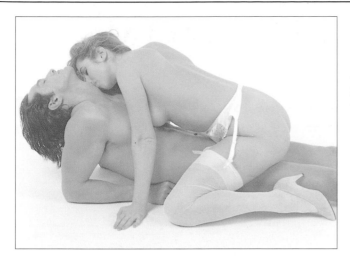

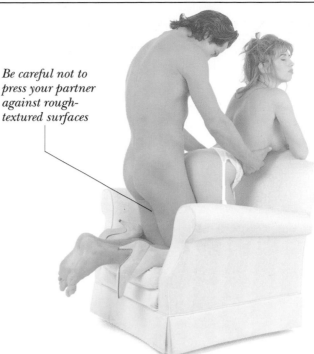

Be careful not to
press your partner
against rough-
textured surfaces

DO IT ON THE FLOOR   Move the furniture out of the
way and make love on the carpet or floor. The hard
surface makes a change from the resilience of a bed, and
if there is enough room you can experiment with all
kinds of different positions.

MAKE LOVE IN AN ARMCHAIR   A large, sturdy
armchair offers you the opportunity to make love in
several positions. For instance, you can both kneel on it,
the woman can kneel or bend over with the man
standing behind her, or he can sit with her on his lap.

*Closing your eyes helps you
savor the sensation, but
watching your partner's
moves will increase your
erotic stimulation*

*Use the floor's sturdy
surface to push off*

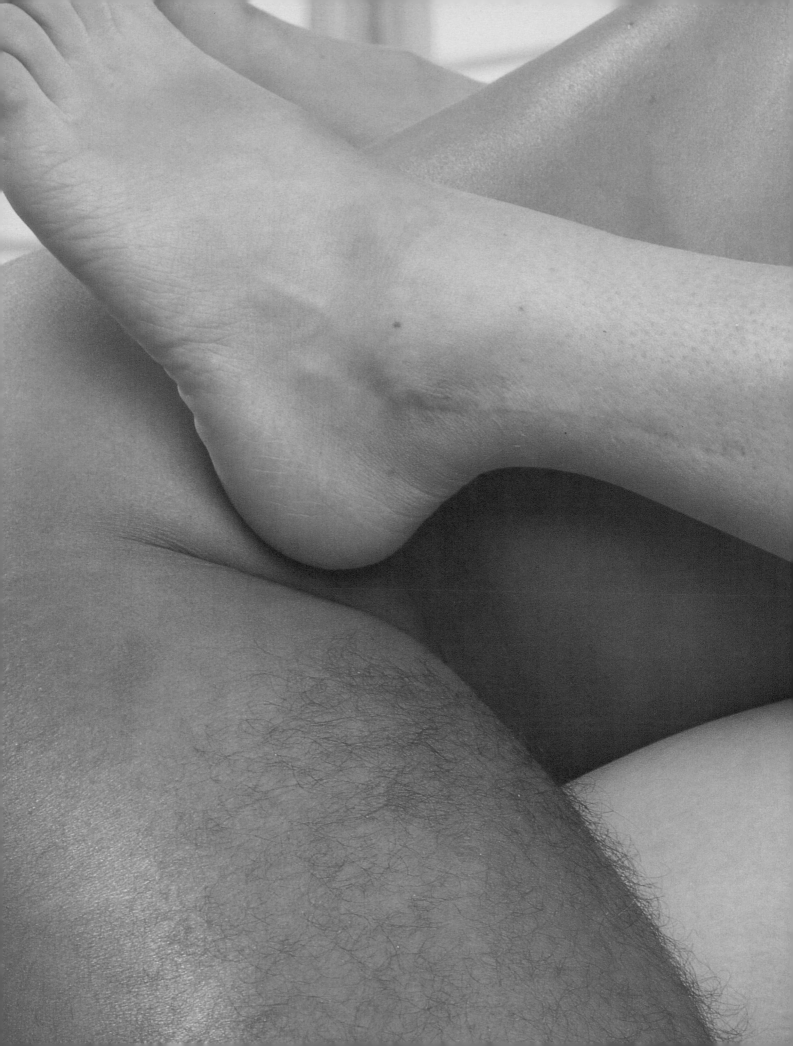

CHAPTER 11

GIVING HIM A SENSUAL MASSAGE

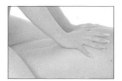

Massage can lay the foundations for relaxation, but once the quality of the touch itself is changed — from using a firm hand to fingertip skimming, from working on the whole body to touching tantalizingly around the genitals — the experience shifts from relaxation to arousal. (For the basic massage strokes, see pages 60-63.)

LEGS AND BACK Begin the session with your partner lying face down, and sit astride his legs. Use warm massage oil to make your hands and his skin slippery and sensuous, and start by leaning back and drawing your hands along the soles of his feet and over his ankles and calves. Then work up from his thighs to his neck.

Use all the basic massage strokes, first firmly, then with relaxed pressure, and finally with light fingertip pressure

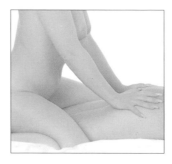

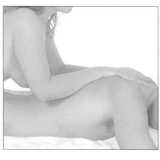

LOWER BACK Using gentle, erotic pressure, work your hands slowly up from his thighs and buttocks to his lower back.

UPPER BACK Pay special attention to the muscles between his shoulder blades and at the base of his neck.

If your bed is too soft, put a comforter or folded blankets on the floor and give your massage there

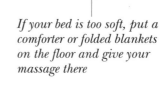

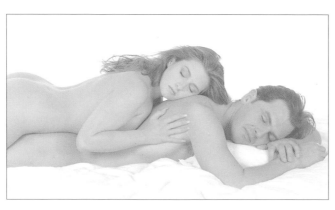

BODY CONTACT When you have finished massaging his back and shoulders, lean forward on to him and slowly and sensuously slide your body from side to side against his. Tighten your thighs against his, and rub your breasts softly across his back.

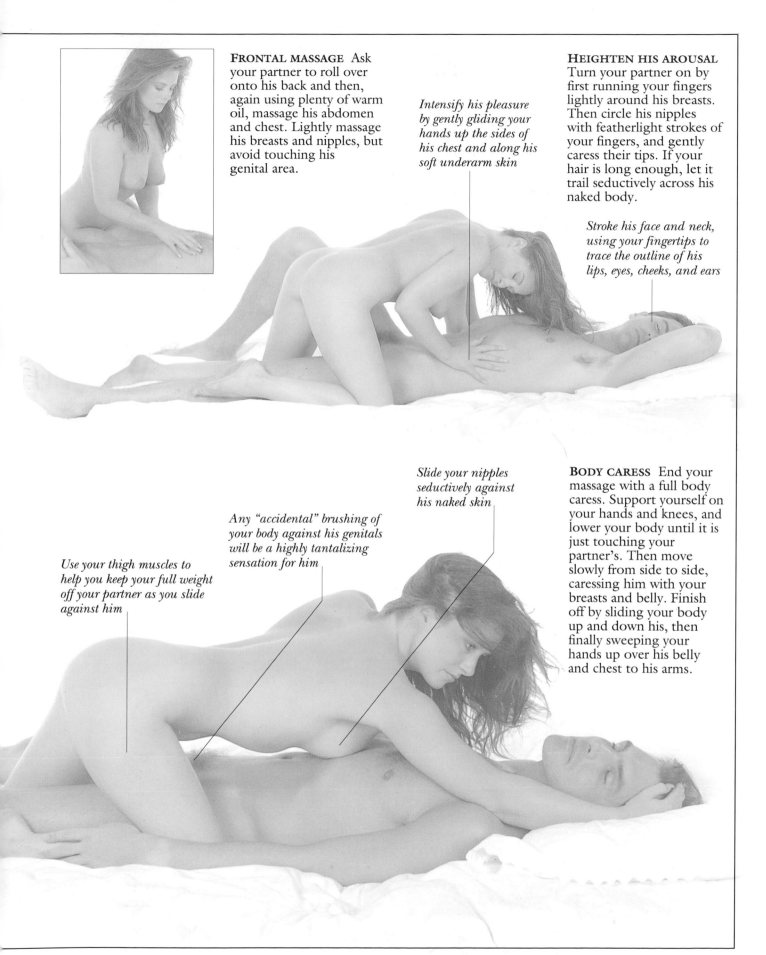

FRONTAL MASSAGE Ask your partner to roll over onto his back and then, again using plenty of warm oil, massage his abdomen and chest. Lightly massage his breasts and nipples, but avoid touching his genital area.

Intensify his pleasure by gently gliding your hands up the sides of his chest and along his soft underarm skin

HEIGHTEN HIS AROUSAL Turn your partner on by first running your fingers lightly around his breasts. Then circle his nipples with featherlight strokes of your fingers, and gently caress their tips. If your hair is long enough, let it trail seductively across his naked body.

Stroke his face and neck, using your fingertips to trace the outline of his lips, eyes, cheeks, and ears

Slide your nipples seductively against his naked skin

Any "accidental" brushing of your body against his genitals will be a highly tantalizing sensation for him

Use your thigh muscles to help you keep your full weight off your partner as you slide against him

BODY CARESS End your massage with a full body caress. Support yourself on your hands and knees, and lower your body until it is just touching your partner's. Then move slowly from side to side, caressing him with your breasts and belly. Finish off by sliding your body up and down his, then finally sweeping your hands up over his belly and chest to his arms.

GIVING HER A SENSUAL MASSAGE

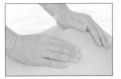

Giving your partner a loving, sensual massage will reinforce the bonds of love between you, and it will be a highly erotic experience for both of you. Make yourselves comfortable in a warm, draft-free room, and if your bed is too soft put a comforter or folded blankets on the floor and give her your massage there. (For details of the basic massage strokes, see pages 60-63.)

START AT THE BUTTOCKS
The female buttocks are rich in nerve endings, so they are highly erogenous. Using warm massage oil to make your hands and her skin slippery and sensuous, lightly run the flats of your hands across each of her buttocks.

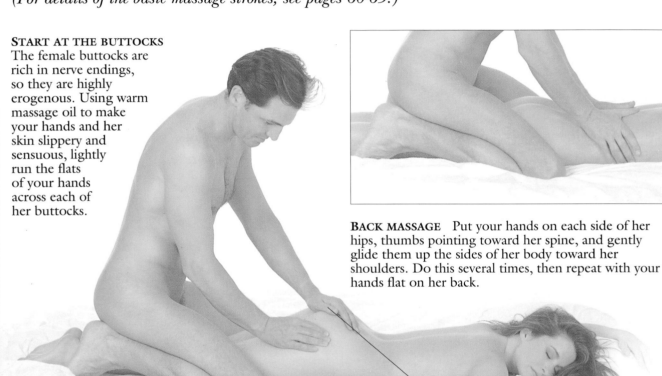

BACK MASSAGE Put your hands on each side of her hips, thumbs pointing toward her spine, and gently glide them up the sides of her body toward her shoulders. Do this several times, then repeat with your hands flat on her back.

Use all the basic massage strokes, first firmly, then increasingly lightly until your fingertips are just brushing her skin

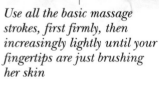

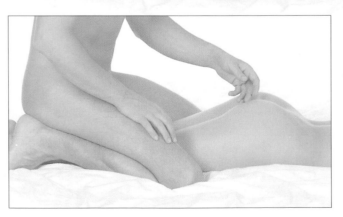

INNER THIGHS Using well-oiled fingers, stroke firmly up the inside of each thigh in turn, from just above the knee up to the buttocks and back. Use only the lightest of finger pressure on the return strokes.

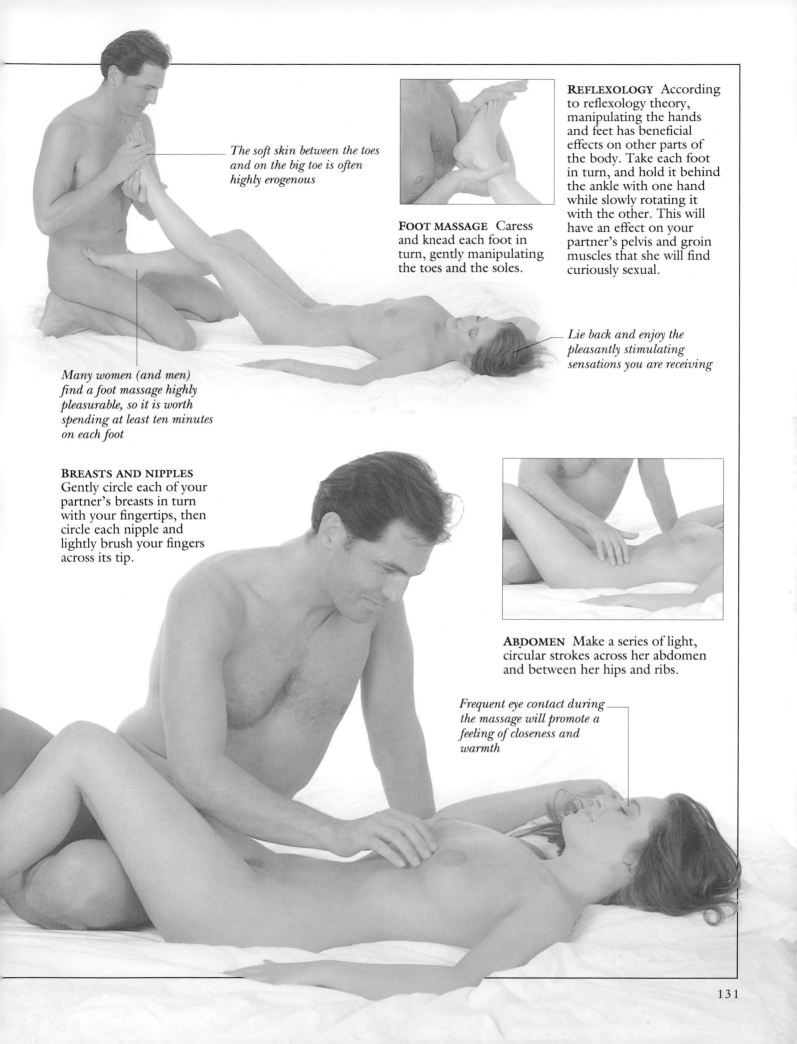

The soft skin between the toes and on the big toe is often highly erogenous

FOOT MASSAGE Caress and knead each foot in turn, gently manipulating the toes and the soles.

REFLEXOLOGY According to reflexology theory, manipulating the hands and feet has beneficial effects on other parts of the body. Take each foot in turn, and hold it behind the ankle with one hand while slowly rotating it with the other. This will have an effect on your partner's pelvis and groin muscles that she will find curiously sexual.

Lie back and enjoy the pleasantly stimulating sensations you are receiving

Many women (and men) find a foot massage highly pleasurable, so it is worth spending at least ten minutes on each foot

BREASTS AND NIPPLES Gently circle each of your partner's breasts in turn with your fingertips, then circle each nipple and lightly brush your fingers across its tip.

ABDOMEN Make a series of light, circular strokes across her abdomen and between her hips and ribs.

Frequent eye contact during the massage will promote a feeling of closeness and warmth

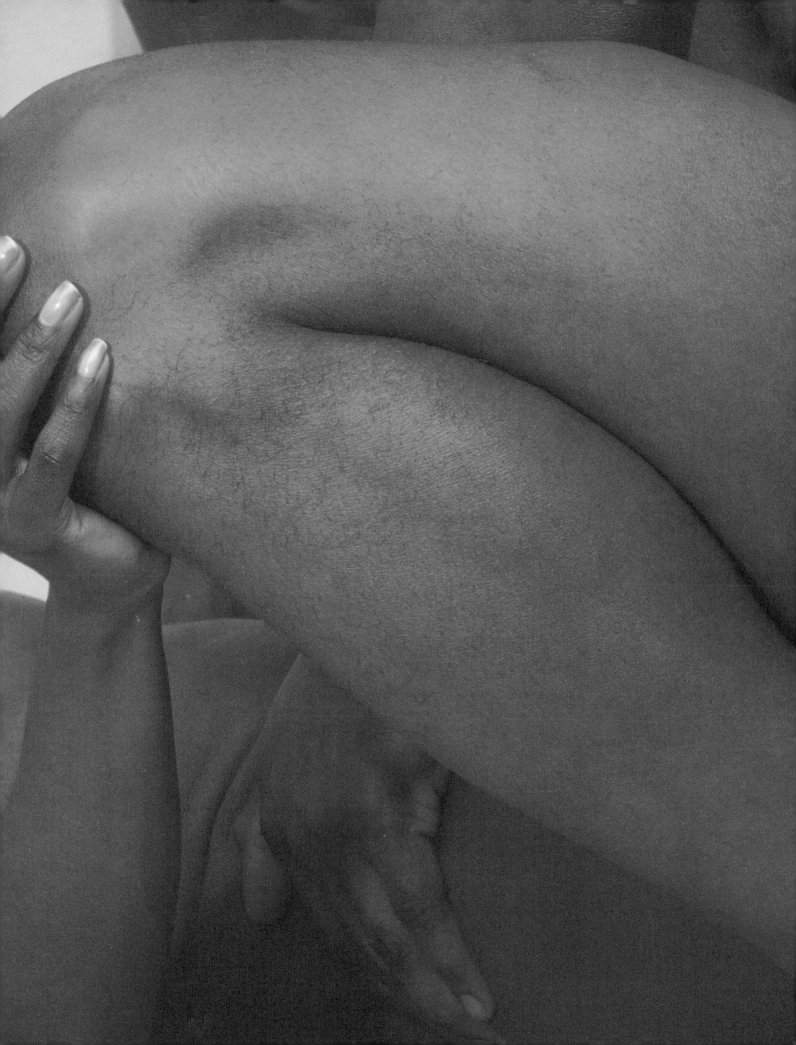

CHAPTER 12

HOW CAN WE EXPLORE OUR DEEPEST FANTASIES?

"Not everyone has sexual fantasies, but many of those who don't fantasize are capable of learning."

SEXUAL FANTASY is regarded by some as a marriage rescuer and an enhancer of eroticism, by others as an escape from reality and politically undesirable. The latter attitude ignores the fact that judicious use of fantasy can be of great value. It can, for example, help some women to experience a climax when they have never been able to do so before.

The use of fantasy allows couples to explore their imaginations and transform lovemaking into a sexual adventure fully involving minds and emotions as well as their bodies.

There is thought to be a link between an individual's sex drive and the likelihood of him or her having sexual fantasies, with people who have a high sex drive being more likely to use fantasy than those with lower sex drives.

In addition, those whose upbringing has conditioned them against sexual feeling, and who thus through guilt have learned to suppress their sex drives, will be less likely to have sexual fantasies

However, the good news is that we can all learn how to overcome such inhibitions and enjoy the erotic potential of our imaginations.

CASE STUDY *Joyce & Neil*

Both Joyce and her partner, Neil, understood the usefulness of sexual fantasy in a relationship, and both of them wanted to introduce it into their sexual activities. But their problem was that neither of them knew how to mention this secret desire to the other.

Name:	JOYCE
Age:	27
Marital status:	DIVORCED
Occupation:	POOL ATTENDANT

Joyce was a pretty but indecisive woman who worked part-time at her local swimming pool. She had a two-year-old son, and was trying to decide on a suitable educational program to improve her career prospects.

"I was married for eight years to a man who simply couldn't turn me on," she said. "His particular brand of sexuality just didn't tune into my erotic wavelength and the marriage eventually fell apart. After that, I had brief, unsatisfactory relationships with two other men and then ended up with Neil.

"Neil is imaginative, very good in bed, gives me wonderful oral sex, and gets me further in the direction of climaxes than anyone else has ever managed, but I have never had a climax with him. I know I can have them because I can get them through masturbation and fantasy. I feel sure sex could really work with Neil, I'm so far along the path with him now, but somehow or other I need him to bring fantasy into it. I really don't have a clue where to start. Do I just ask him? How would he know what I mean? Is there any way in reality in which he can somehow enter my fantasies, or am I just kidding myself?"

Name:	NEIL
Age:	30
Marital status:	SINGLE
Occupation:	ILLUSTRATOR

Neil was a short, dark illustrator who painted lyrical pictures of knights and dragons and of women warriors fighting orcs and trolls. His work was much in demand for science fiction book covers and calendars.

"I think Joyce is one of the sexiest women I've ever encountered," he said. "Yet she is only just beginning to understand that. She has yet to be awakened sexually. What she really needs is some kind of romantic yet directly erotic scenario, and what I'd really like to do is to pretend she has been tied down by a cruel guardian with ropes and left there vulnerable to me. I think this could be wonderful for both of us but I'm terrified of blowing it. I don't want to take the risk of overstepping the mark. What can I do?"

THERAPIST'S ASSESSMENT

When Joyce and Neil discussed their problems with me individually, it soon became clear that what they both wanted was to enhance their sexual activities by the use of fantasy, and that the only thing that stopped them from doing so was the fact that neither knew how to raise the matter with the other. But once they were able to discuss it freely, they were soon confiding and acting out sexual fantasies, and Joyce was climaxing regularly and easily.

Difficulties of communication can sometimes put up the greatest barrier to a special sexual activity which, ironically, both partners may desire. Asking for something out of the ordinary is not easy; to do it successfully you need to take risks, yet give reassurance at the same time.

UNSPOKEN SIGNALS
You also need to read a partner's unspoken signals very carefully. One reason these can be misinterpreted is because your own desire for a particular activity is so great that you project interest onto a partner when it is not necessarily there. The only way to find out who longs for a certain sexual activity is by talking. Ask questions at a neutral time, not when you are poised over your partner complete with thigh boots and whip. Choose a relaxed time for asking these intimate questions — for example, when you are lazing on the grass on a hot summer's afternoon, or during a long car journey.

ASKING QUESTIONS
When asking questions, avoid doing so in an accusatory fashion. Don't say, "You look as if you might get off on a little mild spanking in bed." Instead, use a more indirect approach, such as, "I get the feeling you might like it if I spanked you very lightly when we make love next time. What do you think?" And if you are very uncertain indeed about how your partner might receive even such a tentative question, you could precede that by saying, "There's something sexual I really want to talk about, but I'm finding it very hard. I'm afraid you might get the wrong idea about me."

Most partners, on hearing this, will want to know what it is that is so difficult and will offer reassurance. You can then follow up the reassurance by saying, "This is just a question and won't change anything we already love doing together in bed. But ..." There is no avoiding the fact that you are taking risks by broaching the subject — but on the other hand, if you never do this, you will never progress in your erotic life at all.

ENACTING HIS FANTASY

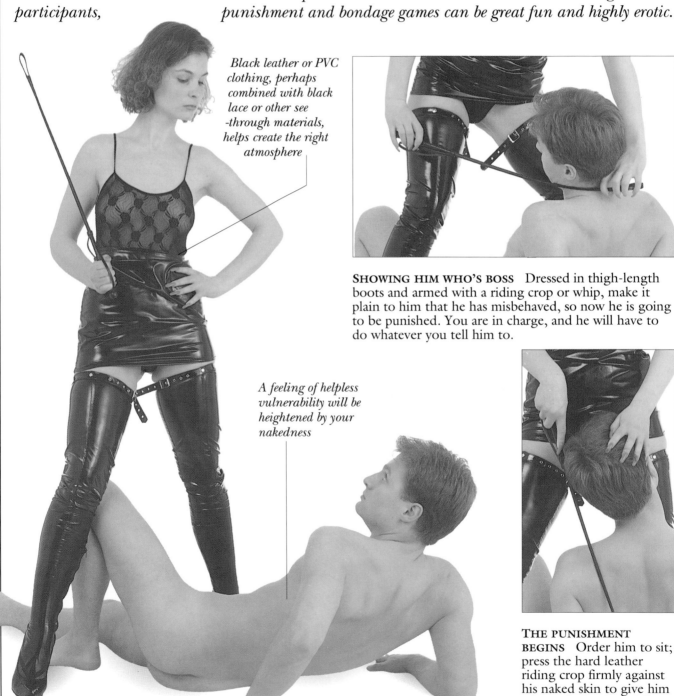

Sexual horizons are broadened most easily by using fantasy to accompany your lovemaking or masturbation. Without having to resort to new partners, you can experience, if only in your mind, an entire range of arousing activities. Punishment and bondage are among the more common types of male fantasy, as evidenced by the number of advertisements that appear offering "discipline" or "correction" services to male clients. Provided that both partners involved in such activities are willing participants, punishment and bondage games can be great fun and highly erotic.

Black leather or PVC clothing, perhaps combined with black lace or other see-through materials, helps create the right atmosphere

A feeling of helpless vulnerability will be heightened by your nakedness

SHOWING HIM WHO'S BOSS Dressed in thigh-length boots and armed with a riding crop or whip, make it plain to him that he has misbehaved, so now he is going to be punished. You are in charge, and he will have to do whatever you tell him to.

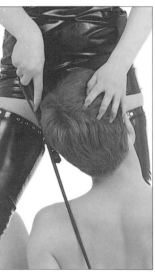

THE PUNISHMENT BEGINS Order him to sit; press the hard leather riding crop firmly against his naked skin to give him a hint of what is to follow.

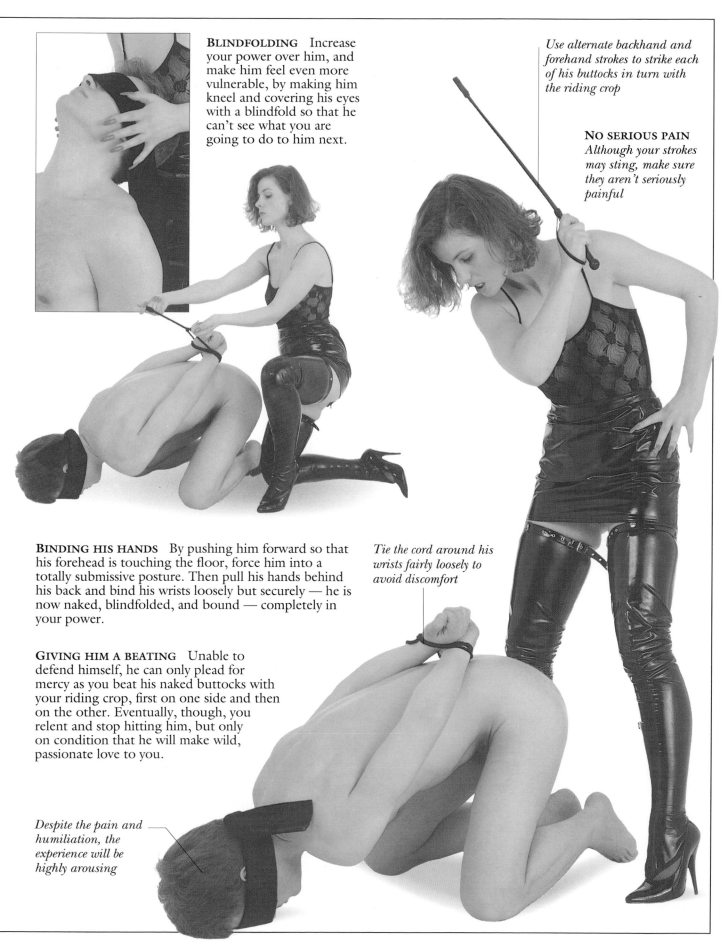

BLINDFOLDING Increase your power over him, and make him feel even more vulnerable, by making him kneel and covering his eyes with a blindfold so that he can't see what you are going to do to him next.

Use alternate backhand and forehand strokes to strike each of his buttocks in turn with the riding crop

NO SERIOUS PAIN Although your strokes may sting, make sure they aren't seriously painful

BINDING HIS HANDS By pushing him forward so that his forehead is touching the floor, force him into a totally submissive posture. Then pull his hands behind his back and bind his wrists loosely but securely — he is now naked, blindfolded, and bound — completely in your power.

Tie the cord around his wrists fairly loosely to avoid discomfort

GIVING HIM A BEATING Unable to defend himself, he can only plead for mercy as you beat his naked buttocks with your riding crop, first on one side and then on the other. Eventually, though, you relent and stop hitting him, but only on condition that he will make wild, passionate love to you.

Despite the pain and humiliation, the experience will be highly arousing

139

ENACTING HER FANTASY

As a way of introducing variety into your sex life without undue effort or threat to an existing relationship, unexpected sexual behavior can be a real turn-on. Women often use the fantasy of a secret lover, occasionally coupled with a feeling of helplessness, to induce increased ardor. A male partner often finds that this type of fantasy, acted out, helps liberate unknown desires within himself as well.

HEIGHTEN ANTICIPATION
If the woman is naked and her partner remains clothed, tension is already created by her seeming vulnerability. Literally being kept in the dark prevents her from anticipating his unexpected caresses, or seeing what he may be doing behind her back.

Gently cover her eyes and be as soft in your movements as possible so as to induce feelings of eroticism, not fear

Rough textures against smooth skin will encourage a variety of feelings, both real and imagined

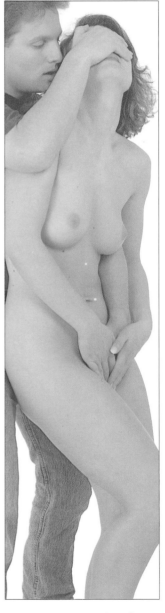

BE SUGGESTIVE Speak in a low voice and tell her what you are going to do with her and what she will have to do for you. Try to keep humor and levity at bay.

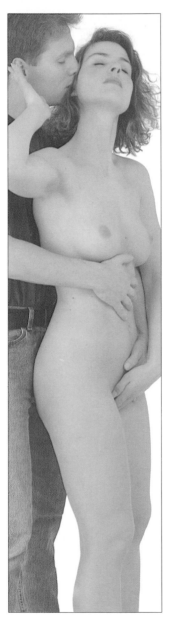

ENCOURAGE HER When she begins to respond to your suggestions, ease up by freeing her eyes, and begin to let your lips and hands caress her body.

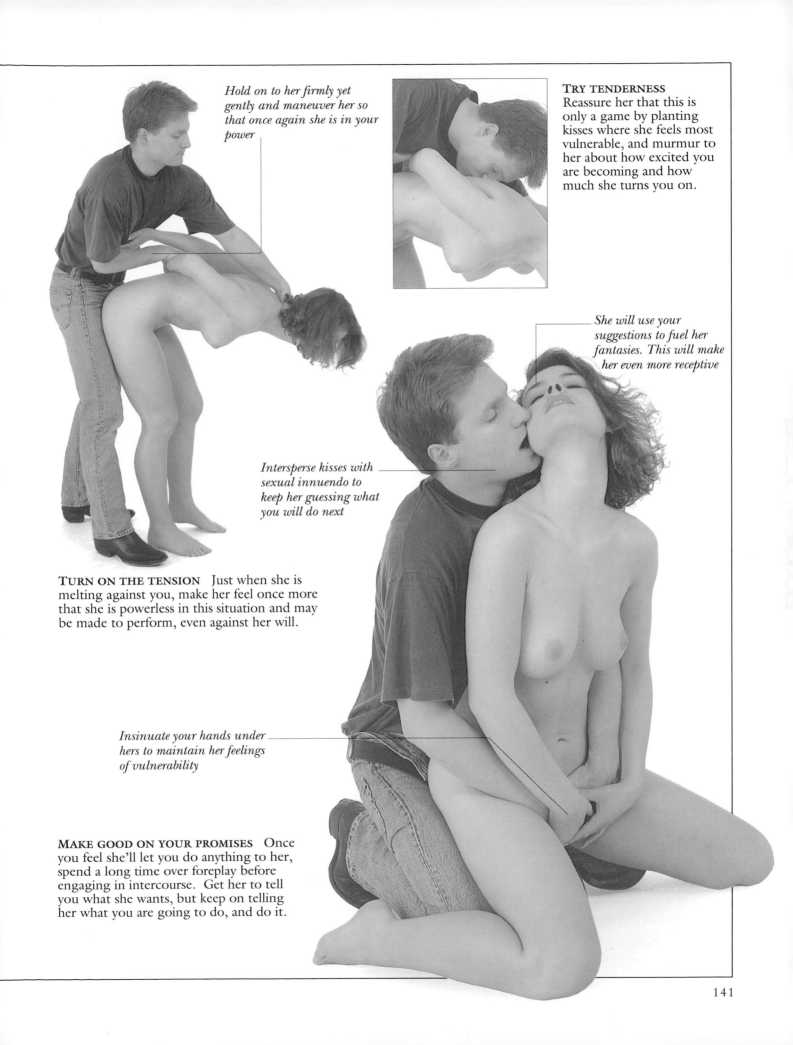

Hold on to her firmly yet gently and maneuver her so that once again she is in your power

TRY TENDERNESS
Reassure her that this is only a game by planting kisses where she feels most vulnerable, and murmur to her about how excited you are becoming and how much she turns you on.

She will use your suggestions to fuel her fantasies. This will make her even more receptive

Intersperse kisses with sexual innuendo to keep her guessing what you will do next

TURN ON THE TENSION Just when she is melting against you, make her feel once more that she is powerless in this situation and may be made to perform, even against her will.

Insinuate your hands under hers to maintain her feelings of vulnerability

MAKE GOOD ON YOUR PROMISES Once you feel she'll let you do anything to her, spend a long time over foreplay before engaging in intercourse. Get her to tell you what she wants, but keep on telling her what you are going to do, and do it.

PLAYING THE INNOCENT

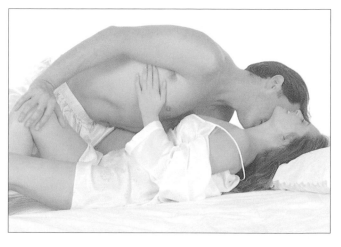

Both a mastery of sexual techniques and a lack of experience are powerful stimulants of sexual desire for both sexes. Women often fantasize about a sexually adroit partner or about initiating a younger man into sex, while men occasionally like an aggressive partner who has them at their mercy but usually prefer to see themselves as the more experienced partner in any relationship. Rediscovering the excitement of "first time" sex is an easy way to put an edge on sexual feelings.

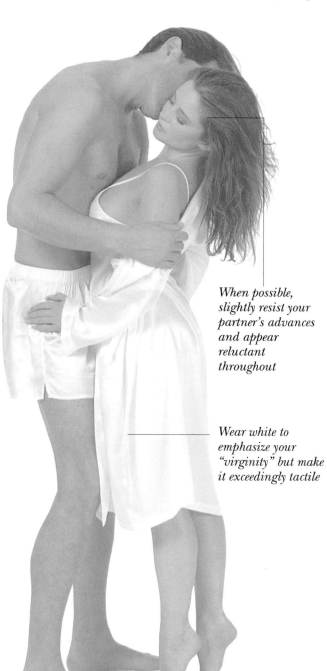

When possible, slightly resist your partner's advances and appear reluctant throughout

Wear white to emphasize your "virginity" but make it exceedingly tactile

LET YOUR PARTNER TAKE THE LEAD Pretend this is your first sexual experience. Simple gestures of affection are permitted, but don't be too overt in your receptivity.

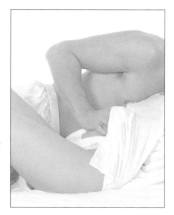

TAKE THINGS SLOWLY Gestures should be long, lingering, and languorous — the slower the movement, the more erotic and arousing it will feel. Your body must be treated as though it were undiscovered territory.

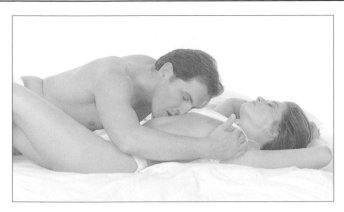

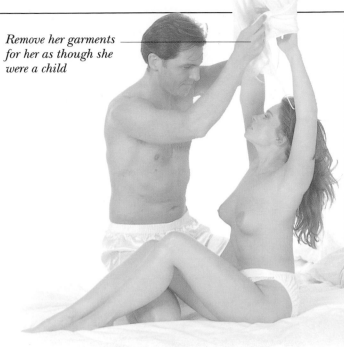

Remove her garments for her as though she were a child

USE A VARIETY OF CARESSES   Use your mouth and hands up and down your partner's body, listening for the responses that tell you she is enjoying what you do.

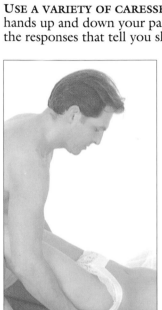

SLIP THINGS OFF   As you remove each garment, ease it off in a nonforceful way yet one that is charged with sensuality.

REMOVE HER GARMENTS ONE AT A TIME   Don't be in too much of a hurry to strip your partner naked. Intersperse removing her garments with gentle caresses as each new part is revealed.

GIVE HER REASSURANCE As you make love to your partner, tell her how good you will make her feel and how she is going to enjoy the experience. Never mind that you've made love to her a hundred times before; this is the first time all over again.

Adopt an on-top position so that she is cradled underneath

Manipulate your partner's body to suit you

Press your legs up against her so that she feels enclosed by you

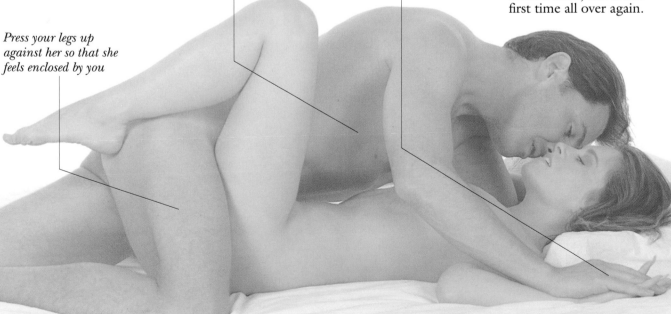

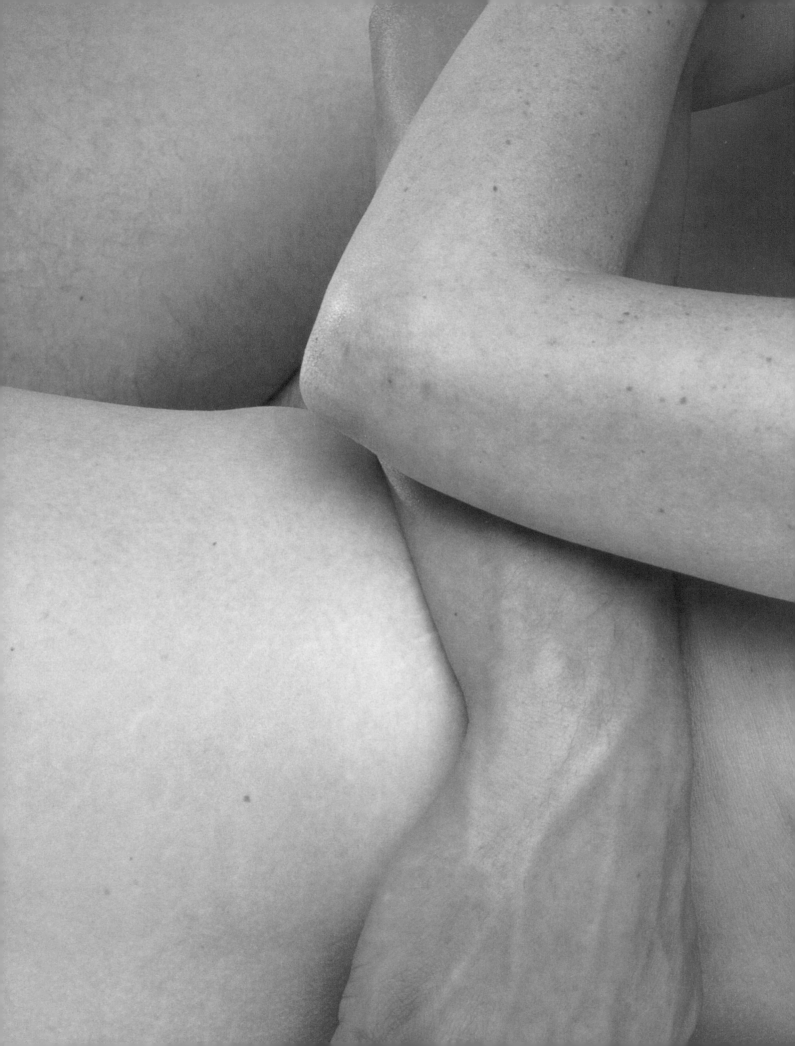

CHAPTER 13

THE SENSUAL CONDOM

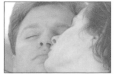

The condom is not only an effective form of contraceptive, it also acts as a barrier to infection with sexually transmitted diseases such as syphilis, gonorrhea, chlamydia, and HIV — putting on a condom correctly can thus sometimes mean the difference between safety and sickness. Some couples, however, are reluctant to use condoms because they think that interrupting their lovemaking to put one on is unromantic and unerotic. But by following a few simple rules, a woman can turn the mundane act of slipping a condom onto her partner's penis into a truly erotic experience.

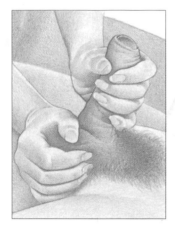

CHOOSING CONDOMS
As a general rule, avoid unknown brands and always check the expiration date on the package. Avoid the strangely shaped condoms with knobbly edges and clitoral ticklers — although they heighten the sensation they are, alas, generally unsafe because they do not fit the penis tightly enough and so may slip off or allow semen to leak into the vagina during intercourse

START WITH A GENITAL MASSAGE   To make the donning of the condom as erotic an experience as possible, begin by treating your lover to a brief but sensuous genital massage.

When slipping a condom onto your lover's penis, use slow, sensuous movements to make the occasion as erotic as possible

MASTURBATE HIM
Change your hand action from genital massage to gentle masturbation of him as a preliminary to slipping the condom onto his penis.

Make putting on a condom part of foreplay; don't wait until your excitement gets the better of you

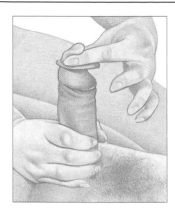 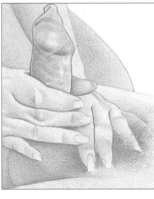 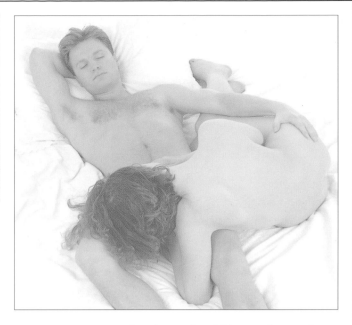

SQUEEZE OUT THE AIR
Gently press the tip of the condom between thumb and forefinger to ensure it contains no air — an air bubble could cause it to split during intercourse.

PUT ON THE CONDOM
Put it on the tip of his penis with one hand and roll it down to the base with the other. If he is uncircumcised, first push back his foreskin.

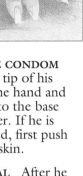

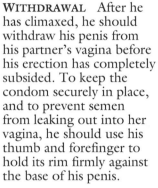

WITHDRAWAL After he has climaxed, he should withdraw his penis from his partner's vagina before his erection has completely subsided. To keep the condom securely in place, and to prevent semen from leaking out into her vagina, he should use his thumb and forefinger to hold its rim firmly against the base of his penis.

USING CONDOMS Condoms should be used to make oral sex safe (above) as well as to provide protection during intercourse (below). For oral sex, use flavored condoms to make the act of giving fellatio through a condom more enjoyable for her.

You may find that using a condom helps you to maintain your erection longer and delays ejaculation

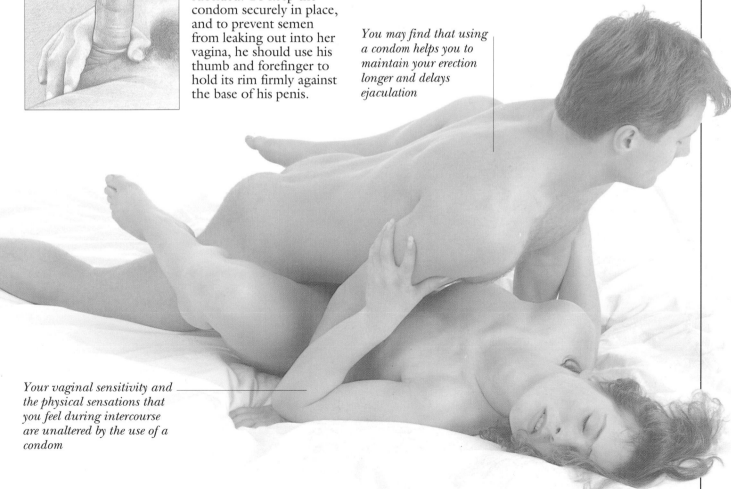

Your vaginal sensitivity and the physical sensations that you feel during intercourse are unaltered by the use of a condom

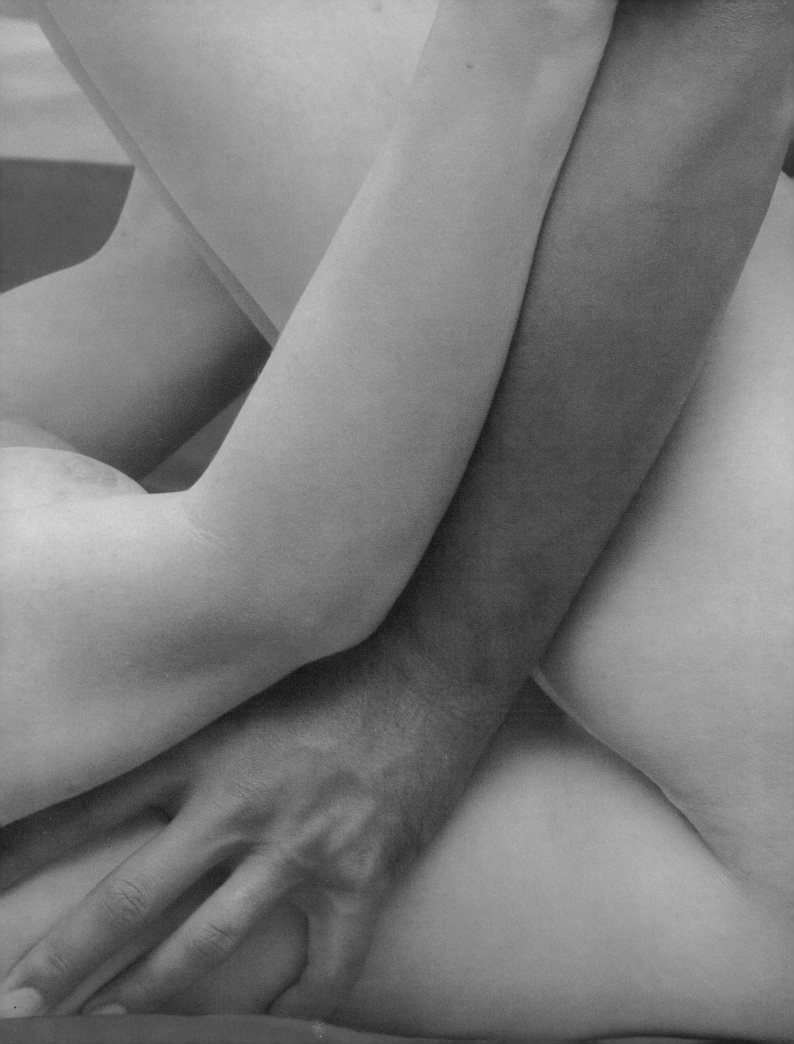

CHAPTER

14

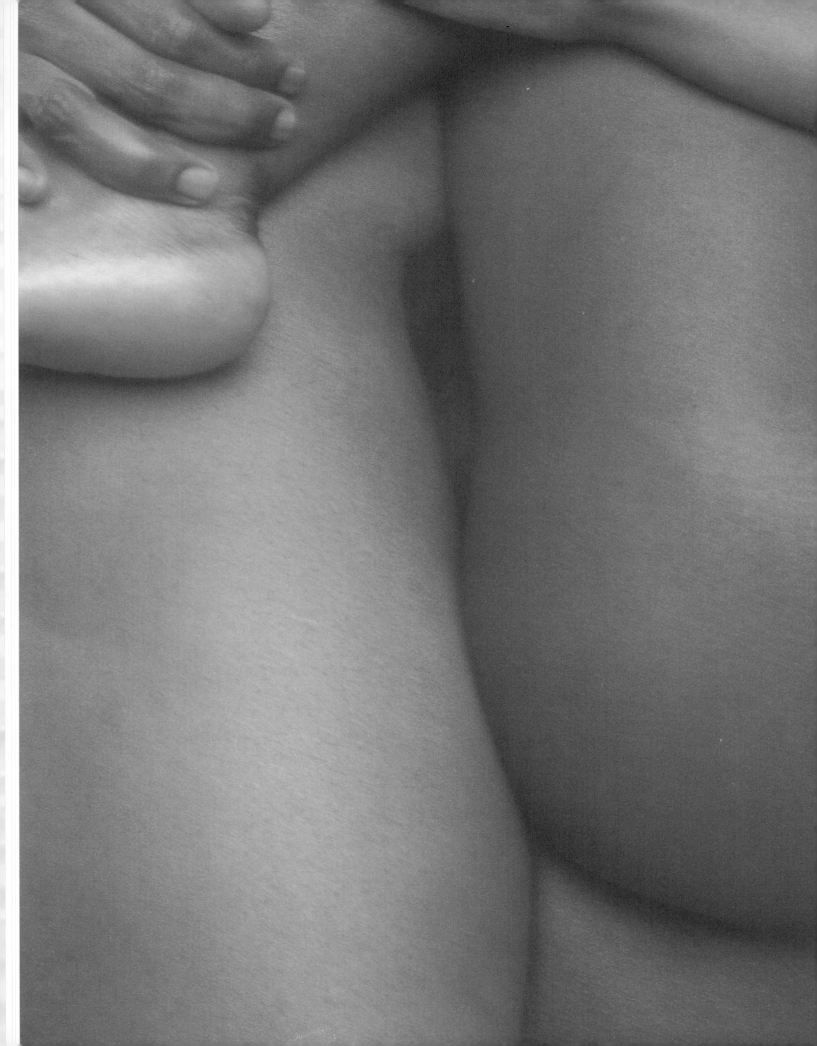

CHAPTER 15

LOVEMAKING ON A CHAIR

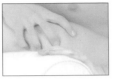

Even something as potentially exciting as sex can become boring. By making love on a chair instead of in bed, you can try out a wide range of different lovemaking positions, and perhaps add some welcome variety to your sex life. As a bonus, many of these positions leave your hands free, allowing you to exchange caresses.

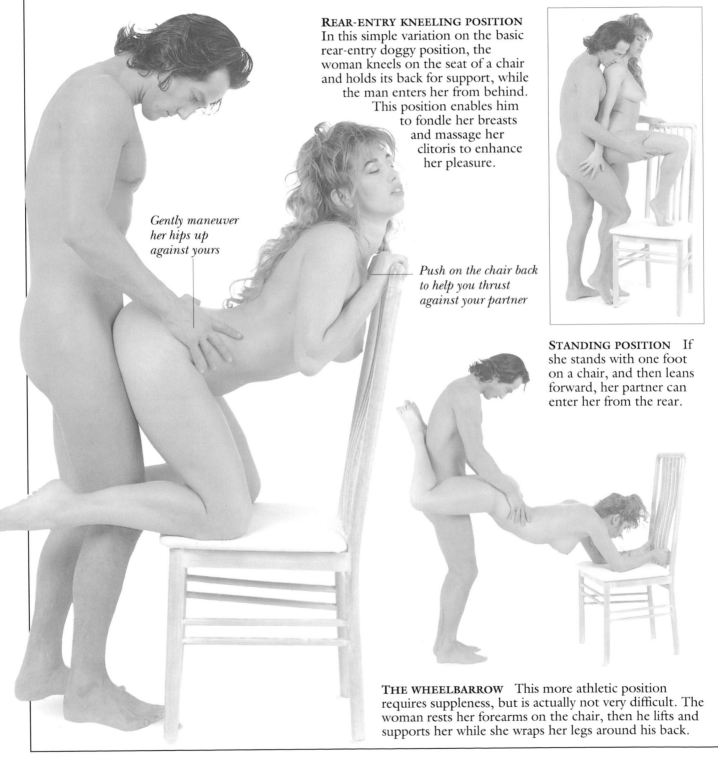

REAR-ENTRY KNEELING POSITION
In this simple variation on the basic rear-entry doggy position, the woman kneels on the seat of a chair and holds its back for support, while the man enters her from behind. This position enables him to fondle her breasts and massage her clitoris to enhance her pleasure.

Gently maneuver her hips up against yours

Push on the chair back to help you thrust against your partner

STANDING POSITION If she stands with one foot on a chair, and then leans forward, her partner can enter her from the rear.

THE WHEELBARROW This more athletic position requires suppleness, but is actually not very difficult. The woman rests her forearms on the chair, then he lifts and supports her while she wraps her legs around his back.

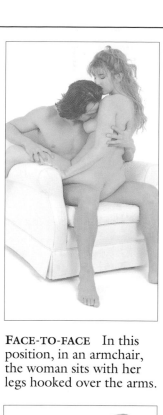

FACE-TO-FACE In this position, in an armchair, the woman sits with her legs hooked over the arms.

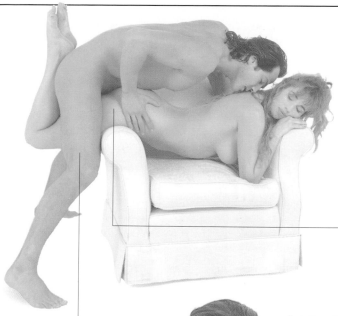

ACROSS THE CHAIR ARM
When the man has entered her from the rear, the woman gently closes her legs to enhance his sensations. Alternatively, she can keep one foot on the floor and extend the other leg back between his as far as she can.

Savor the different sensations that are aroused when she varies the positions of her legs

Position yourself so you can enter her without causing discomfort

Let the stimulating sight of your partner reaching orgasm excite you further

Use your hands to raise and lower yourself

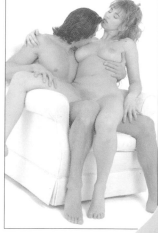

REAR-ENTRY POSITION
The woman sits on her partner's lap and is almost sideways.

LYING ON HIS LAP To get into this position, the woman starts by sitting on the man's lap and facing him. When he has entered her she leans back, supported by his hands, until she is lying along the tops of his thighs.

175

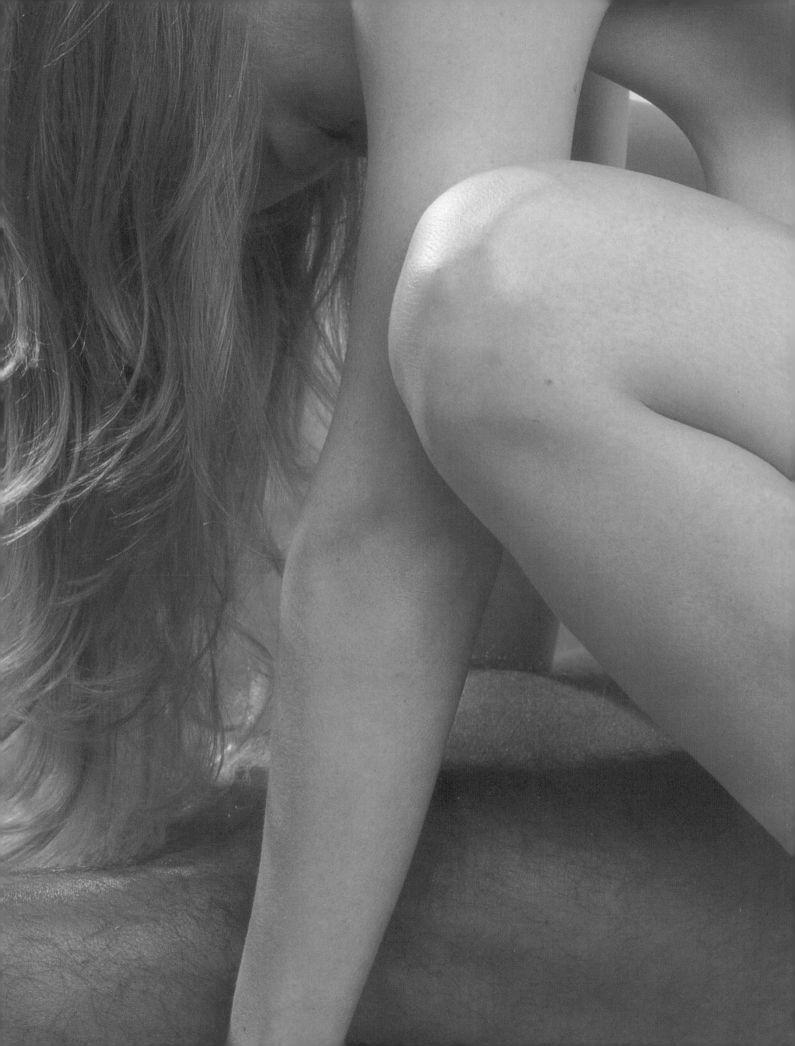

CHAPTER 16

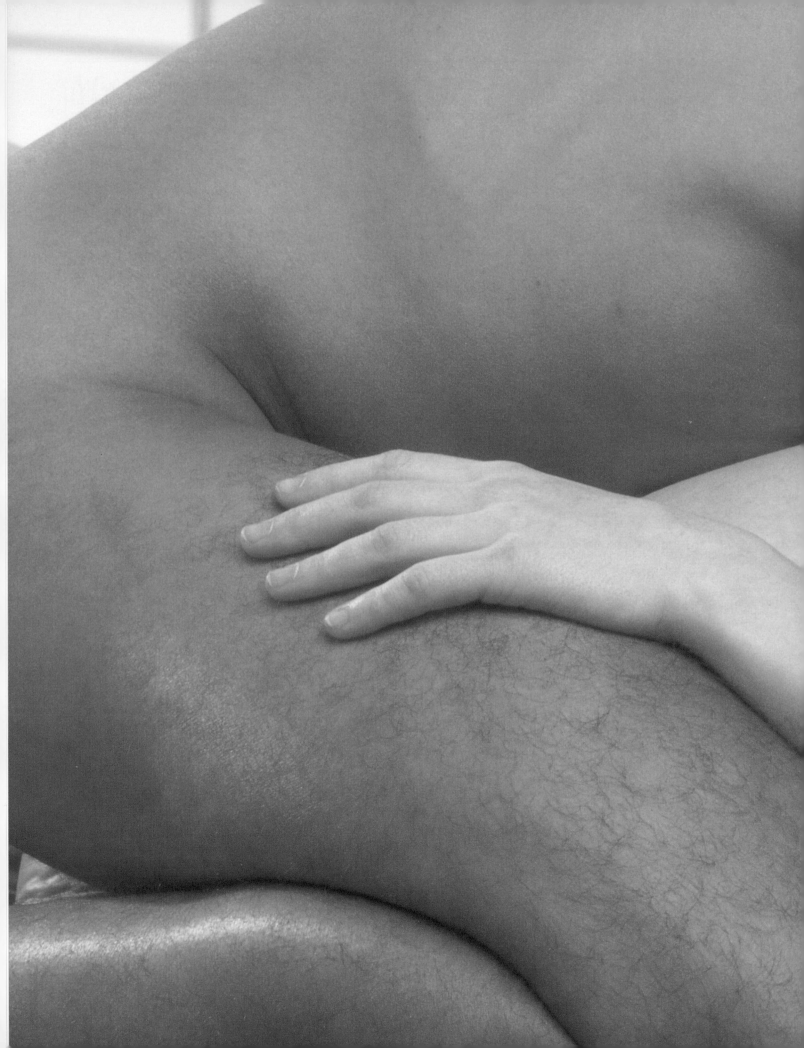

CHAPTER

17

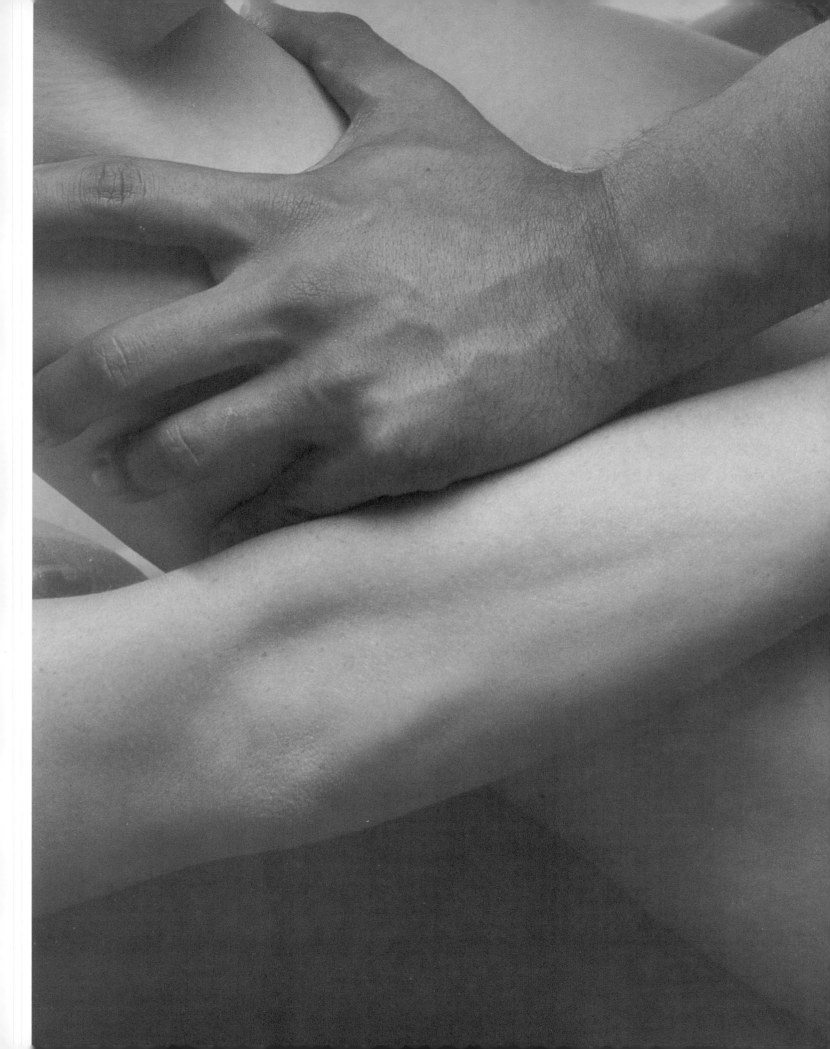

CHAPTER

18

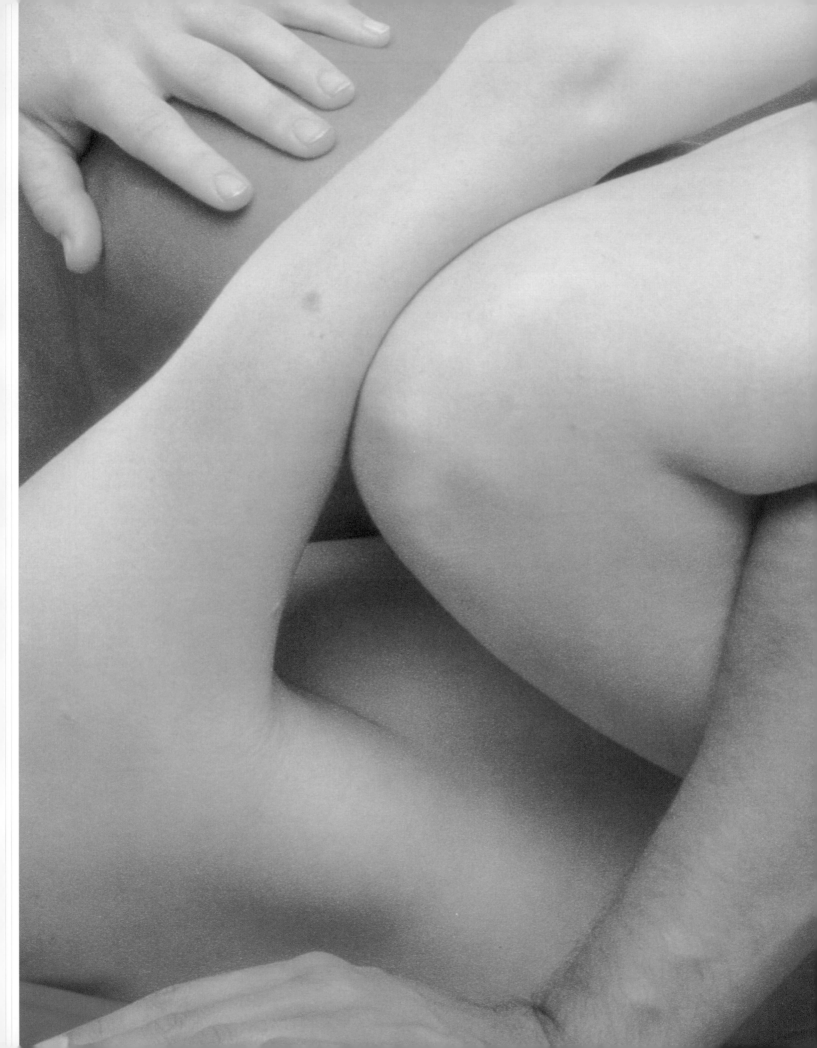

CHAPTER 19

HOW CAN WE BRING BACK DESIRE?

"Even when desire has dwindled away almost to nothing, if both partners really want to rekindle it — then there are ways it can be done."

THE ONE single ingredient that has proved to be the most difficult to quantify in human sexual response is the desire of one individual for another.

What exactly is sexual desire? How do we get it? Is it something caused by our hormones or is it a psychological phenomenon, or is it perhaps a combination of both of these factors? Why doesn't it last? And when it fades away, as it so often does, how can we get it back?

These are all questions that sex researchers have been asking for years, but they have yet to come up with any completely satisfactory answers to them.

More importantly, they are also questions that are asked by ordinary men and women who love each other but, without really knowing why, are finding it hard to raise the enthusiasm for making love to each other.

CASE STUDY *Jan & Elaine*

Jan and Elaine's long and loving marriage was showing signs of strain because Jan, despite his love for his wife, had lost interest in making love to her and no longer got the thrill from sex that he once did. This left Elaine feeling undervalued. And since the children were grown up and had left home, she had started to think about leaving him and finding a new lover.

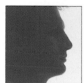

Name:	JAN
Age:	45
Marital status:	MARRIED
Occupation:	SERVICE MANAGER

Jan was a tall, thin, graying man with tortoiseshell glasses, a sharp stare, and a charming smile. He had come to this country as a young refugee, married young, and had two grown-up children.

"I had very precarious beginnings in this country," he said. *"I arrived at the age of ten, with parents who had nothing. But in spite of doing well — first in school, then with my career — I still felt insecure until I met Elaine. She gave me an almost physical sense of relief. With her, my fears vaporized. Now, it feels as though she's part of me. I love her and there's no way I want the marriage to end.*

"But in the past few years our sex life has declined. It has gotten harder and harder to make the effort. Admittedly, when I have done so, usually because Elaine has become frantic, it's been as wonderful as ever. But I just don't get that sense of need for her body anymore, and I don't get the buzz out of sex I used to."

Name:	ELAINE
Age:	47
Marital status:	MARRIED
Occupation:	SYSTEMS ANALYST

Elaine, youthful-looking with soft red hair, a slim, willowy figure, and an obvious zest for life, was stylishly dressed and managed to look glamorously sexy.

"He's not the only one who's concerned," she told me. *"I'm sure I ought to rid myself of the belief that sex represents love, and therefore Jan doesn't love me anymore — I can see that logically this doesn't follow. But underneath I'm feeling more and more unloved. As I see it, the problem isn't on my side. I still desire Jan. I still try to initiate sex. And once every few months I finally goad him into doing something about it. But that isn't enough, and I'm thinking of just giving up. I'm reaching a dangerous age. My kids have left home. My career is blossoming again, and although I haven't been tempted yet, I can see, so easily, how women fall in love with other men under these circumstances."*

THERAPIST'S ASSESSMENT

Nobody knows what makes lovers lose desire for each other. The cause could be familiarity, or resentment over past hurts, or the changing appearance of a lover as the years pass. Or it could be because of parenthood, or seeing a spouse as a companion or sibling rather than a lover. The list goes on and on.

The options for people in Jan and Elaine's situation are straightforward. They can separate with great pain and form new partnerships, which may indeed restore their joie de vivre. They can remain together but tacitly agree to condone each other's affairs elsewhere. They can continue as they have been doing but with the danger that the marriage will become so stagnant it will die of inertia. Or they can take a shot at reviving the sensual side of life together. This doesn't guarantee orgasms, but it does mean that the partners learn to build up the amount of time they spend on sensual enjoyment. This goes a long way toward reviving warmth and tenderness.

MEDICAL PROBLEMS
There are occasionally medical or hormonal reasons why men and women lose desire, and naturally medical advice should be sought if this is the case. But both Jan and Elaine were in good health, so they decided to try to learn new tactile skills together, giving themselves an attractive common platform of sensuality.

WEEKLY EXERCISES
They agreed to embark on a weekly series of exercises, starting with mental self-examination to reveal their inner fears and desires. The second week's exercise was mutual physical self-examination (see pages 80-83) and that was followed by regular weekly touch sessions, at first with intercourse forbidden but, as time passed, eventually including it.

SELF-HELP THERAPIES
There are two other therapy models that couples can consider to assist themselves with solving the problem of waning sexual desire. The first is the sexual enhancement program (page 60) and the second is the three-day Tantric program (see page 202). The emphasis in both of these is in building up tactile pleasure without, at first, a sexual imperative, so that sensuality becomes a strong bond once more between the lovers, and a sound basis upon which desire can be rebuilt.

My program for
REKINDLING DESIRE

The dampening or death of desire may be countered by experience of a different order. Tantric philosophy, which holds that through sex we can experience expanded and enhanced being, can offer new sexual vistas. Tantra, like yoga, originated in India; nicknamed the "science of ecstasy," it heightens and prolongs the special rapport that exists between a man and a woman during lovemaking. The point of the exercises practiced over this three-day program is to aim consciously at merging yourself ecstatically with your partner and, through him or her, with the rest of the world. If that sounds like a tall order, it's worth remembering that in your mind, anything is possible.

If you were a devoted student of Tantric philosophy, you would have to go through an extensive program of training your senses to detect subtle nuance and change. You would practice physical exercises to strengthen the muscles needed to make extended intercourse a pleasure rather than a pain, and explore mental exercises to extend your imagination. In this way you would train yourself to be aware of not only your own feelings but also those of the man or woman with whom you wish to become one. The three-day program described here is not as rigorous as a full Tantric program, but it will help bring you and your partner closer together and to re-awaken your desire for each other.

THE FIRST DAY The object of the first day of the program is to get you and your partner to relax and talk freely and candidly about yourselves and your relationship. You should be completely open with each other, but avoid saying anything hurtful.

On the first day you both remain clothed and close physical contact is restricted

SEXUAL CONTINENCE The three-day program comes with a strict rule about sexual continence: there will be no intercourse or orgasm until the latter part of the third day. It is best carried out away from your everyday circumstances, preferably somewhere quiet, private, comfortable, and in the countryside, so that the beauty of the surrounding scenery enhances the experience.

Read the instructions for each day while lying close together, and do your best not to give way to longings that lead to coupling — some of the practices can be deeply arousing. But since the Tantric ideal is to prolong the entire sex act so that it becomes greatly enhanced, there is method in this abstinence.

You may hold hands, but you should not kiss or caress each other

Stage THE FIRST DAY

The first day of the three-day program is a day for getting to know each other. No matter that you may have lived together for ten years: today you will begin to tear aside the veil of privacy that, over the years, you have instinctively but unconsciously placed between yourself and your lover, and you will dare to expose yourself without reservation.

After a light breakfast, go for a walk in the beautiful countryside where you are staying. Enjoy the scenery and the peace and quiet, and try to relax and forget about the problems of your everyday life. Spend the time talking, and reminisce about what it was like when you first met. Remember the beauty of your love in the beginning, the way you felt about each other in those early days of your relationship, and the things you did together.

OPEN UP When you talk with your partner about yourself and your relationship, let down your defenses and be completely open about your feelings. Don't be afraid to show emotion: hold hands, laugh, cry, and talk freely of your fears, fantasies, hopes, and hates. Speak of anything and everything — but do not say anything that might hurt your partner.

For example, if you discuss a former lover or partner, stress that the affair is over and done with, and don't talk about it too regretfully because that might give your partner the impression that he or she is some kind of second best. And if you decide to mention that you find fault with something about your partner, hasten to add that the fault is really a minor one and that his or her good points far outweigh the bad ones.

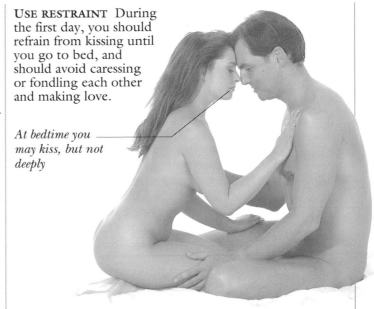

USE RESTRAINT During the first day, you should refrain from kissing until you go to bed, and should avoid caressing or fondling each other and making love.

At bedtime you may kiss, but not deeply

Give each other plenty of time to speak and to express opinions, thoughts, hopes, and fears, and pay attention to what is said. Make each other feel good, and do caring things like making each other little gifts.

USE RESTRAINT Although you may hold hands, or walk arm in arm, that should be the extent of today's touching. Hold back from kissing, fondling, and making love. In the evening, talk a little more. Share your feelings about this exercise and its progress, and talk about what it is like to be together without making love.

When you go to bed on the first night, kiss if you must, but not deeply, and do not caress. Sleep in each other's arms, but hold back from caressing and lovemaking. There is plenty of time ahead in which to make love.

NO INTERCOURSE On the first night, sleep in each other's arms if you can do so comfortably, but do not fondle or caress each other and avoid intercourse — abstinence will intensify your feelings.

The spoons position is a comfortable one for sleeping closely together

Put your arms around your partner, but do not caress or fondle

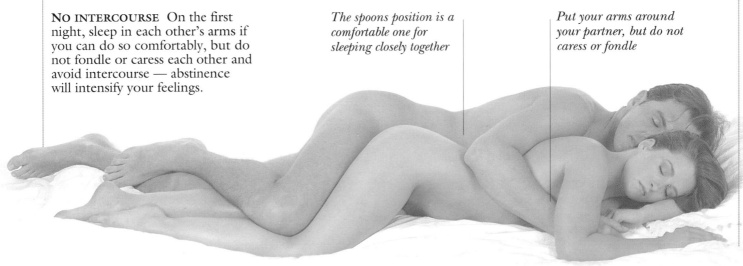

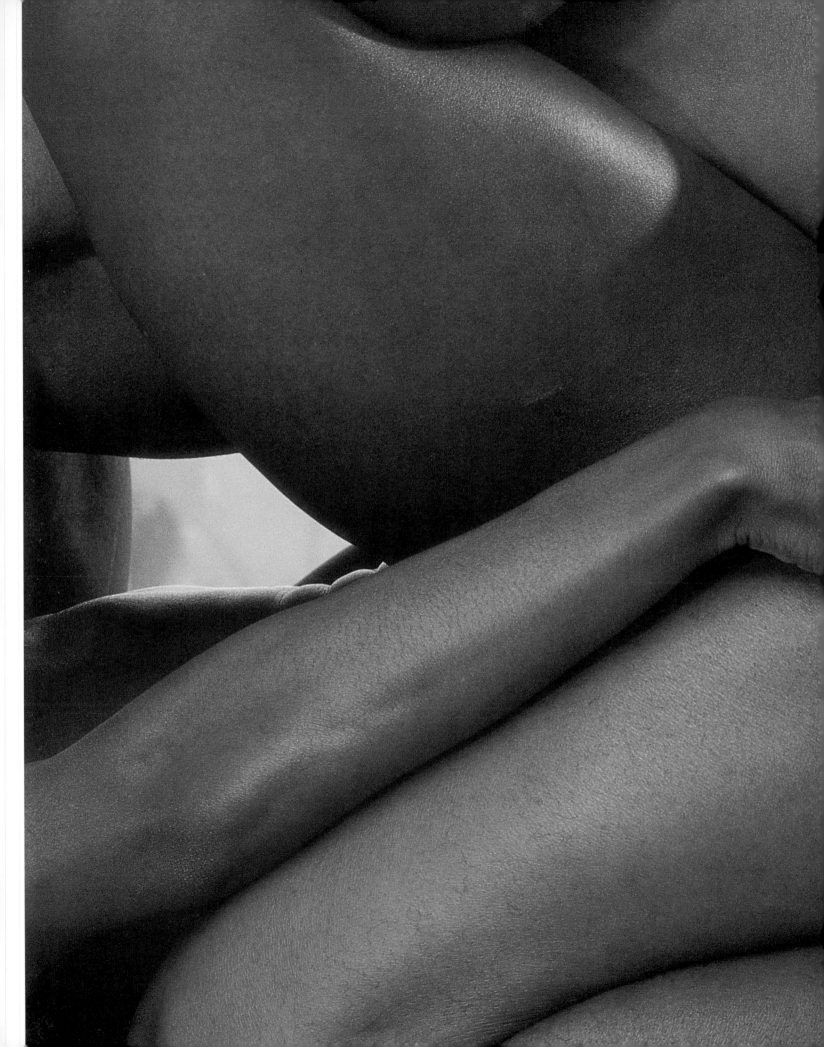

CHAPTER

20

THE PATH OF SEXUAL TAO

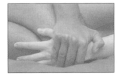

The Ancient Chinese reveled in the vigor and ardor of young lovers. Instead of dismissing the sex activities of birds and beasts as diminishing the human spirit, they actually encouraged young lovers to look and learn from the natural behavior of animals. The pure raw sensuality of the wild tiger or even the domestic donkey were to be sought after and embraced. The same "chi" that flows through man and woman also flows through all of life, and so, far from seeing creatures as objects to be disliked and dismissed, humans were taught to seek and channel the same vigorous energy.

SPRING DONKEY

With the woman kneeling down on her hands and knees, the man positions himself at the woman's hips; he grasps them and inserts his penis. The man should experiment with shallow and deep thrusts, trying faster and slower speeds. This position frees partners from having to support each other's body weight, while allowing the man to caress the woman's thighs, back and breasts. In China, donkeys often mate in spring, which is how this position got its name.

WHITE TIGER

The woman crouches forward, resting on her forearms, with her legs bent at the knees and held shoulder-width apart. The man then lies on top of her, using one hand to hold her neck while inserting his penis. His thrusts should be a combination of fast and slow. White Tiger was so named because in this position the man moves like a male white tiger.

The man can massage the sensual nerves at the base of his woman's neck as he thrusts

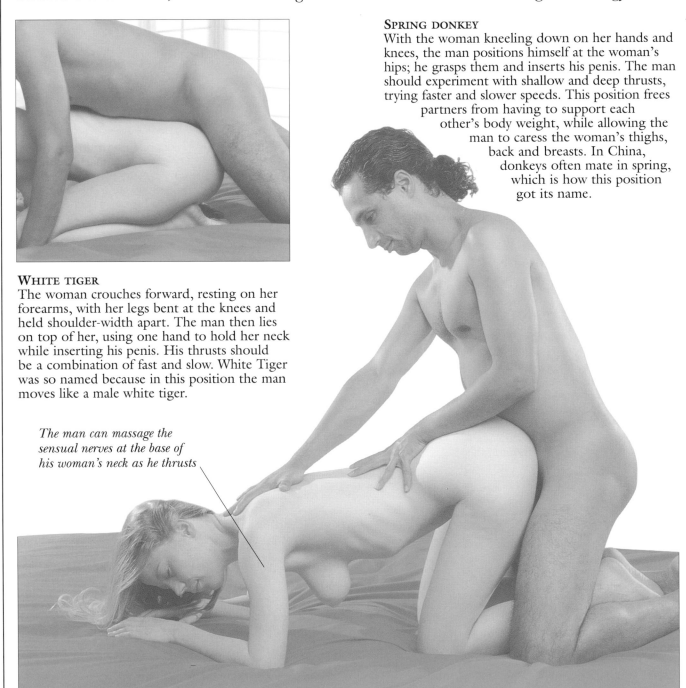

JADE JOINT

The woman lies on her back, bending her legs at the knee and pulling them up to hip level. The man kneels below the woman's hips and inserts his penis. This position enables the man's penis to touch the back of the woman's vagina, and is so named because the couple resemble a jade joint.

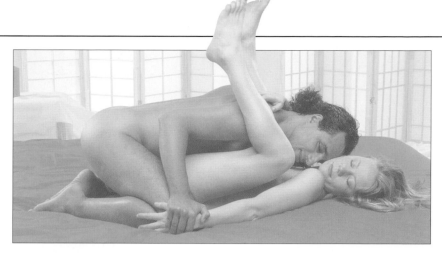

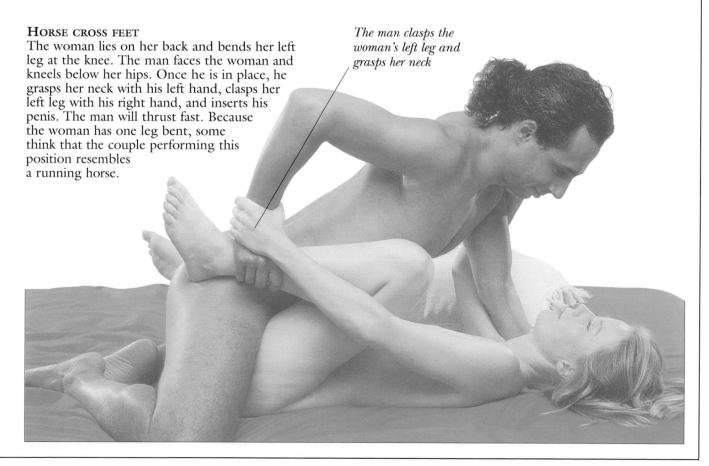

DRAGON TURN

The woman lies on her back with her legs bent at the knees and held against her chest. She holds her feet away from her body. Facing the woman, the man kneels below her hips. Holding her tight, the man inserts his penis, alternating between deep and shallow thrusts. The Dragon Turn is so named because the Chinese believe it resembles the mythical creature, which has long limbs and a flexible body.

HORSE CROSS FEET

The woman lies on her back and bends her left leg at the knee. The man faces the woman and kneels below her hips. Once he is in place, he grasps her neck with his left hand, clasps her left leg with his right hand, and inserts his penis. The man will thrust fast. Because the woman has one leg bent, some think that the couple performing this position resembles a running horse.

The man clasps the woman's left leg and grasps her neck

219

SEX AS HIGH ART

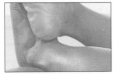 *The fact that sex was seen as healing and pleasurable did not prevent it from also being used as a version of art. The Chinese thought that sex at its best might become a form of beautiful display. In the dance between male body and female form, intricate shapes are formed, by the intertwining of sinuous limbs and the stretch and shudder of rhythmic movement. Out of this creative undulation might flow the shapes and poses of birds and beasts in movement. Capturing movement is never easy on any canvas, but here is one that provides a live display of art in action.*

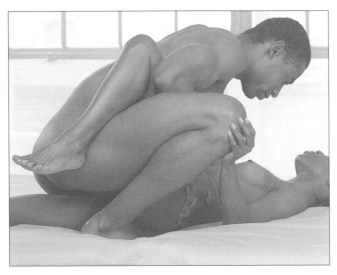

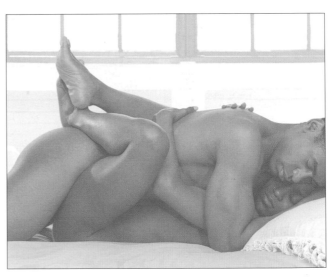

MANDARIN DUCK
The woman lies on her back with her left leg bent and her right leg straight. The man then kneels forward on his right leg with his left leg out behind. He tucks her left leg over his right thigh and inserts his penis. Because they mate for life, mandarin ducks are considered the Chinese lovebirds.

TWO FLYING BIRDS
The woman lies on her back. Facing her, the man lowers himself over his partner, supporting himself with his hands and knees. The man inserts his penis, then the woman wraps her legs over and around the man's buttocks, crossing her feet. The position is called Two Flying Birds because some believe that this is what it resembles.

CICADA
The woman lies face down, raising her hips slightly above the bed. The man, also face down, lowers himself above her, supporting his weight with his elbows and feet. He penetrates her and gently thrusts, being careful to keep the movements shallow. Though the woman's movements are restricted, she still can move her hips to coordinate with the man's movements. The movement of both partners' legs resembles the beating wings of two mating cicadas.

The man must take care not to crush his partner during this gentle stroke

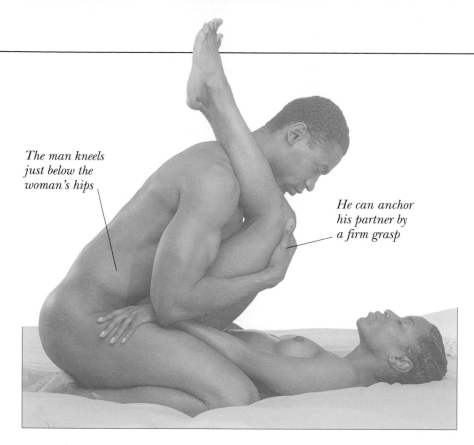

The man kneels just below the woman's hips

He can anchor his partner by a firm grasp

WILD HORSE JUMP

The woman lies on her back. The man faces the woman and kneels below her hips. Once the man is in place, the woman raises her legs and rests her ankles on his shoulders. The woman can hold her hand over the bed post or brace her palm against the wall or headboard to help hold her body steady. The man then holds the woman's thighs, inserts his penis and thrusts hard and fast. With the Wild Horse Jump, the penis is in contact with the back of the vagina. When the woman moves in this position, it almost appears as if she is bucking like a wild horse.

TWO FISH

The couple lies side by side, facing each other. The woman wraps one leg around the man's hip. He inserts his penis, then holds onto her raised leg. Since the length of the man's penis and the depth of the woman's vagina affect each partner's sexual sensations, the man should experiment with both shallow and deep thrusts until finding a type of thrust that suits both individuals. This position is thought to resemble two flounder fish swimming side by side.

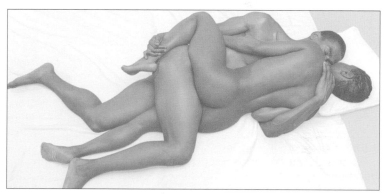

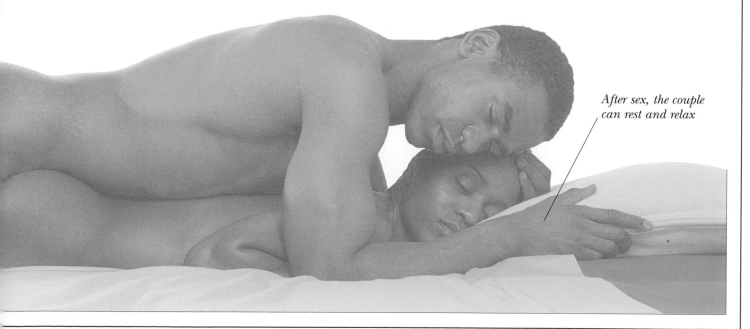

After sex, the couple can rest and relax

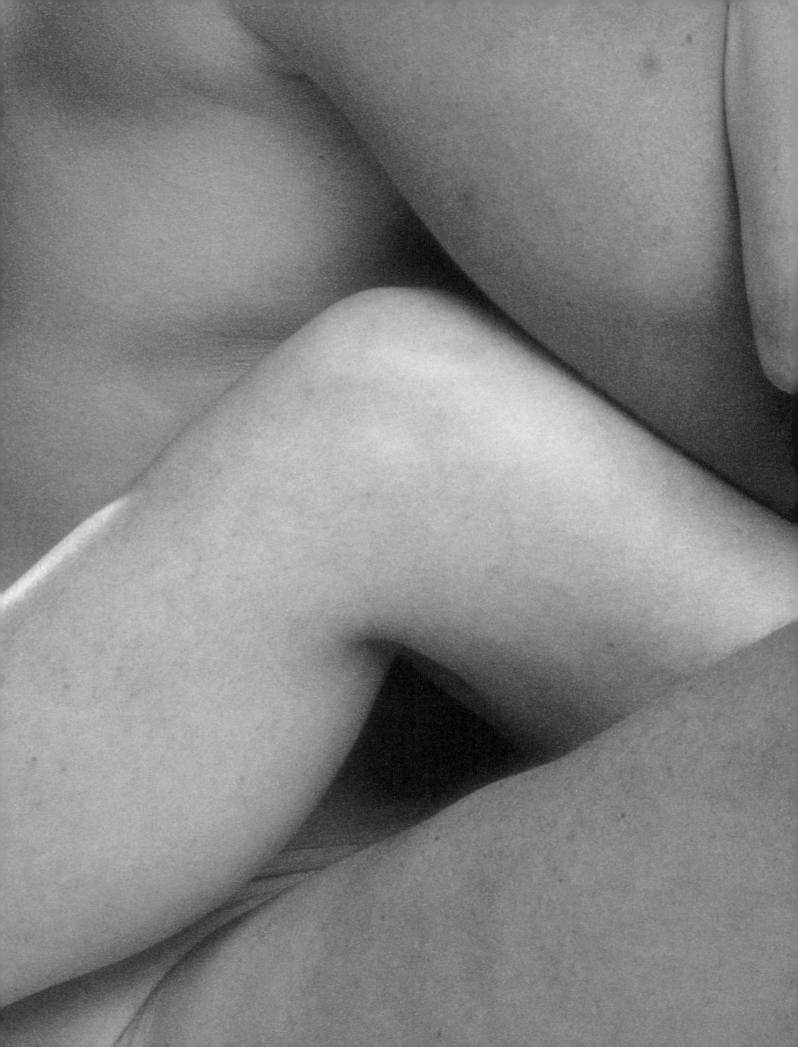

CHAPTER 21

HOW CAN I GET OVER SEXUAL REJECTION?

"One of the most important steps in getting over sexual rejection is to regain confidence in your own sexuality."

REJECTION, whether it happens during the course of a relationship or when one is breaking up, is never easy to cope with. It can lead, on the part of the one who is rejected, to feelings of inadequacy and worthlessness and can make people so afraid of more rejection that they find it hard to form new relationships.

When sexual rejection happens during a relationship, it may be because of simple sexual incompatibility or it may be that one partner rejects the other for reasons not directly connected with sex. For instance, some people reject their partners as a method of punishing them for some real or imagined offense, while others grow to dislike their partners so much that the idea of having regular sex with them becomes unthinkable.

Whatever the reason for it, sexual rejection can be hard to handle, but if it happens to you, there are positive steps that you can take to help you get over it and to restore sexual self-confidence.

CASE STUDY *Diana*

Diana's husband, Monty, to whom she had been married for ten years, had left her for another woman. During their marriage he had often criticized her sexual performance, and when she came to see me she was so lacking in sexual self-confidence that it was holding her back from forming new relationships.

Name:	DIANA
Age:	37
Marital status:	SEPARATED
Occupation:	CHEMIST

Diana was a perfectionist who ran her home and her job meticulously; she had no children, felt very wounded by Monty's rejection of her and, although longing for a new relationship, was scared of risking her emotions again.

"Every time I think about dating a new man, I feel terrified," she confessed. "Even though I keep telling myself it can't be so, I know I must be a complete failure in bed. Monty spent a lot of time telling me how awful I was. How does anyone ever risk finding out what it's like with someone else when the upshot might be to face that again?

"I gave myself heart and soul to Monty, did everything for him and it was just never good enough. And apart from everything else, I still care about him. I actually still want him — God knows how or why. I can't imagine being able to go to bed with anyone else.

"Monty used to accuse me, among other things, of being very passive in bed, and it's true that I was passive with him. But I've often fantasized about doing all kinds of things to a man I've really desired. I honestly think Monty was so critical he frightened me from taking any initiative. I may not be very versatile in bed, but I've always enjoyed sex. Also, I've always had the sneaking suspicion that I might be better at sex with someone who genuinely made me feel good. No one's ever done that. How do I ever let go with someone new after all this? And what do I do with my sex drive?"

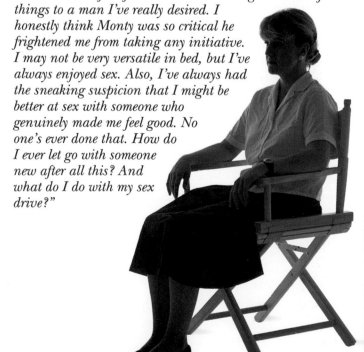

THERAPIST'S ASSESSMENT

There were two components to Diana's problem: her feelings of rejection and sexual inadequacy, and her perfectionism. Perfectionists who set themselves impossible targets make failure unavoidable, and it is always worth looking into a perfectionist's background and figuring out where that need for perfection comes from. In many cases, it turns out to be the result of trying, in childhood, to please a demanding parent for whom the best was never enough.

CONTINUING PATTERN
Even when we leave home, the pattern of trying to please continues, transferred from parent to teacher, lover or boss. Sometimes we may be lucky and feel rewarded by someone who appreciates what we are doing. In this way, we grow to relax and to understand that perfectionism is not vital. More often than not, though, we will have unconsciously picked a partner who feeds into these insecurities and plays on them, probably because they feel familiar — rather like that impossible parent we tried so hard to please.

COUNSELING AND ASSERTIVENESS
Counseling would help Diana to make connections with her belief system in the present and understand how it linked with her childhood. And simple assertiveness (see page 72) would enable her to do what she really felt like doing, without feeling guilty about it, rather than blindly following early patterns.

SEXUAL SELF-KNOWLEDGE
Sexually, Diana needed to find out about herself. She had never masturbated, even as a child, and had only experienced orgasm through intercourse. Possessing a solid background of knowledge about her own sexual responses and sexual interests would give her increased confidence so that when she came next time to a new relationship, she would have more, sexually, to feed into a new love affair.

SEXUAL SELF-PLEASURING
More importantly, through a self-pleasuring routine (see page 226), she could find out how it is possible to be a highly sexual individual without relying on a partner. Of course, masturbation has different emotional dimensions to it than intercourse, but it can be a powerfully arousing and satisfactory experience in its own right.

My program for FEMALE SELF-PLEASURING

Women are brought up and educated to look after others. They are taught to be support systems: mothers, teachers, nurses. With all that caring to do, it can often be difficult for a woman to remember that she deserves to give herself time, too. This self-pleasuring program for women is therefore aimed at helping you to put a little self-indulgent luxury back into your life. Details of a similar self-pleasuring program for men are given on pages 228-229.

Stage 1 THE RAG DOLL EXERCISE

Prepare your surroundings so that they are warm, private, and comfortable. Give yourself at least an hour. Enjoy a warm bath with luxury soaps and sweet-smelling bath oils. (If you are going to use massage oil for the final stage of this program, float the bottle in the bathwater so that it warms up.) Then dry yourself in warm, fluffy towels and do the rag doll exercise to help you relax.

DEEP BREATHING You do the rag doll exercise sitting upright in a comfortable armchair. Breathe deeply, and once you are comfortable with a breathing rhythm, relax your body so that slowly but surely you let it slump over until, finally, you look as limp as a rag doll.

RELEASE TENSION As you slump there limply in the armchair, explore your body for tense spots. If you find any, deliberately tense and relax them until you have eliminated all the muscular tension from your body and you truly feel as though you are made of floppy material. When you have stayed relaxed in that position for at least five minutes, slowly raise first your torso and then your head again, starting from the waist and leaving the head to roll back up into place last.

Stage 2 THE PELVIC LIFT

The pelvic lift is a bioenergetic exercise that enables you to feel energy flow in your thighs and pelvis. It is also a soothing exercise for the relief of tired backs.

Lying on your back, draw your knees up so that your feet are squarely on the floor. Then put your arms along your sides, palms flat down on the floor. Push your abdomen upward and arch your back so that your buttocks are high off the ground. Your body's weight should be supported almost entirely by your shoulders and feet so that you are actually

THE PELVIC LIFT This exercise enables you to feel energy flow in your thighs and pelvis. It is also soothing for tired backs.

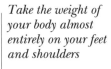

Take the weight of your body almost entirely on your feet and shoulders

resting on your shoulders. Hold this position for a couple of minutes, and then let your body gently down on to the floor again. Lie there on your back for a couple of minutes or so, peacefully relaxing, and then do the squatting exercise.

Stage 3 THE SQUATTING EXERCISE

Squat down with your arms inside your legs and your feet flat on the floor. You will find it isn't easy to maintain your balance doing this, but after a little practice it becomes much easier.

GENITAL RELAXATION The object of the squatting exercise is to open up your genitals and relax them. Breathe deeply, and as you do so, imagine that the breathing is coming from your genitals. Continue for three minutes, then lie on your bed and relax for a minute or two before giving your body and genitals a sensual massage.

SQUATTING EXERCISE
The object of the squatting exercise, which becomes much easier to do after a little practice, is to open up your genitals and relax them.

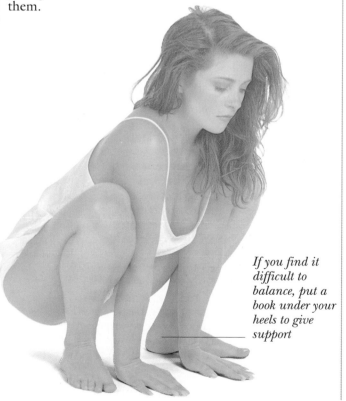

If you find it difficult to balance, put a book under your heels to give support

Stage 4 SELF-MASSAGE

Begin your sensual self-massage, using warm massage oil if you want your hands to feel especially slippery and sensuous, by lying on your back and caressing your arms, shoulders, and thighs. Then run your fingers and hands over your more erogenous zones, such as your breasts, before turning your attention to your genitals, sliding your fingers into and around your vagina, and stimulating your clitoris.

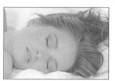

Self-stimulation p232

FURTHER SESSIONS Try to treat yourself to further self-pleasuring sessions at regular intervals. Use these hours of privacy to escape from the pressures of everyday life and to do absolutely anything you want to, provided that it pleases only you — one woman I know of chose to spend her sessions lying naked on a sheepskin rug in front of a roaring fire, listening to lyrical music through headphones while reading an exciting novel.

FEMALE MASTURBATION

Many women use masturbation as a regular and enjoyable part of their sexual activities, but others feel guilty about doing it — usually because they have been told, wrongly, that masturbation is unhealthy or sinful.

• Masturbation, and the urge to masturbate, are now known to be completely natural urges in both men and women. And there is no truth in the old but persistent myth that female masturbation leads to concupiscence (unbridled lust) or to nymphomania.

• That story may have arisen because a woman with a high sex urge is more likely than others to masturbate and to be sexually active, and in less enlightened times such behavior would have made her the target of much sexual innuendo and slander.

• Most women who masturbate regularly use their understanding of masturbation to boost their love lives. If you know you are capable of orgasm, you don't let yourself get put down easily by a partner who is a poor lover, and if you love someone who is inexperienced, you can help him by letting him know what turns you on.

• And you can guess intuitively, from your own knowledge of turn-on, what might appeal to others — although there can be some discrepancy between the sexes here.

My program for MALE SELF-PLEASURING

The basis of the self-pleasuring concept is to learn how to spend time on yourself that is purely for the purpose of pleasure. For those men brought up to believe you should always take care of others first, this can be surprisingly difficult to practice, but self-pleasuring is worth the effort not only for the enjoyment it gives you, but also because it enables you to know your own sexual response and allows you to be a fully functional sexual being regardless of whether or not you have a partner. Details of a self-pleasuring program for women are given on pages 226-227.

Stage 1 RELAXATION

Prepare your surroundings so that they are warm, private, and comfortable. Give yourself at least an hour. Enjoy a warm, relaxing bath, taking your time with sensitively soaping and rubbing yourself. If you are going to use massage oil to make your hands feel slippery and sensuous in the final stage of this program, float the bottle in the bathwater now so that it warms up.

TENSE-AND-RELAX After the bath, make yourself comfortable on a towel on the floor of a warm private room and carry out the tense-and-relax relaxation exercise (page 45).

Stage 2 GROUNDING

Grounding is a bioenergetic exercise that lets you feel in touch with the earth and helps you to sense the energy that flows through both the ground and you. It enables you to feel the power in your body, in particular in your upper legs and pelvis.

BREATH CONTROL Stand with your legs eight inches apart and your knees slightly bent, fists pressing into your back just above your waist. On an in-breath, let your head fall back and at the same time press your heels firmly down into the ground (the floor).

Hold this position for as long as you can bear, breathing regularly but lightly as you do so. When the time comes when you can no longer maintain the position and you have to stand upright, do so on an out-breath.

Once you are standing upright again, pause for a very brief rest. Then let the upper half of your body flop over forward so that the tips of your hands are reaching down and nearly touching the ground. Keep those heels grounded. After a couple of minutes, stand upright again and relax.

You should, after a couple of grounding sessions, start to feel a vibration in the tops of your legs. Once you get this feeling of vibration, you know that the exercise has worked — the energy flow has been released.

MALE MASTURBATION

Contrary to Victorian propaganda, masturbation does not make you blind or deaf, give you the flu, drive you crazy, or kill you. The notion that each teaspoonful of lost semen weakens you to the same degree as giving a pint of blood lost is totally without foundation. Masturbation is a natural and harmless expression of sexuality.

• The fear about masturbation most often voiced to sex therapists is: "If I masturbate, will I get stuck in a pattern of sexual response that won't work when it comes to intercourse?" The truthful answer is that a few people do get stuck because they are inhibited about disclosing their masturbatory activities to a partner, and therefore can never break emotional barriers, which would allow them to relax and climax.

• What about addiction, the other masturbation fear? The only people who are truly addicted to masturbation — they can't leave themselves alone, day or night — are seriously disturbed men and women who are suffering from a form of mental illness and who demonstrate this with unacceptably overt self-stimulation. Masturbation is not the cause here, but the effect.

Stage 3   PELVIC CIRCLING

This bioenergetic exercise helps you to feel energy in your genitals. While standing, move your hips in a circular fashion as if you were hula-hooping. Move your hips first to the right and then to the left, and then eventually weave them in a figure-eight shape. Breathe evenly throughout the exercise.

When you have finished the exercise, lie down on your bed and allow yourself to relax for a minute or two before giving your body and genitals a sensual massage.

GROUNDING This is a bioenergetic exercise that helps you to sense the energy that flows through both the ground and you.

Let your head fall back, breathe lightly, and press your heels into the floor

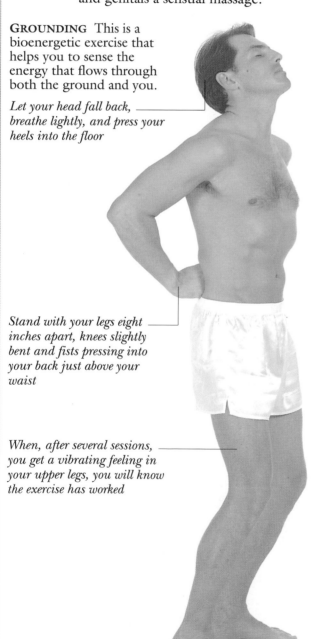

Stand with your legs eight inches apart, knees slightly bent and fists pressing into your back just above your waist

When, after several sessions, you get a vibrating feeling in your upper legs, you will know the exercise has worked

Stage 4   SELF-MASSAGE

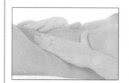

Male stimulation p230

Begin your sensual self-massage, using warm massage oil to make your hands feel especially sensuous, by lying on your back and running your hands and fingers over your arms, shoulders and thighs, including erogenous zones such as your nipples. Then turn your attention to the stimulation of your genitals. At further sessions do anything you want, provided it pleases only you — self-stimulation, reading, watching TV, anything.

PELVIC CIRCLING This bioenergetic exercise helps you to feel the flow of energy in your genitals.

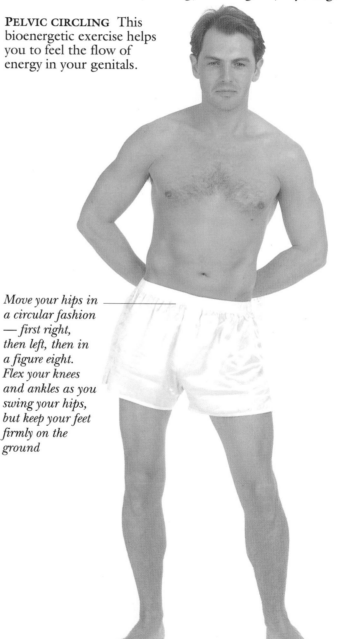

Move your hips in a circular fashion — first right, then left, then in a figure eight. Flex your knees and ankles as you swing your hips, but keep your feet firmly on the ground

MALE SELF-STIMULATION

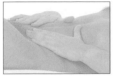

The knowledge of your own body and its sexual responses that self-stimulation teaches you can form the basis of a good sexual relationship with your partner. More importantly, self-stimulation can provide you with a solid sexual foundation upon which you can build up your overall feeling of self-confidence. It can thus help to establish you, in your own eyes, as a man of value.

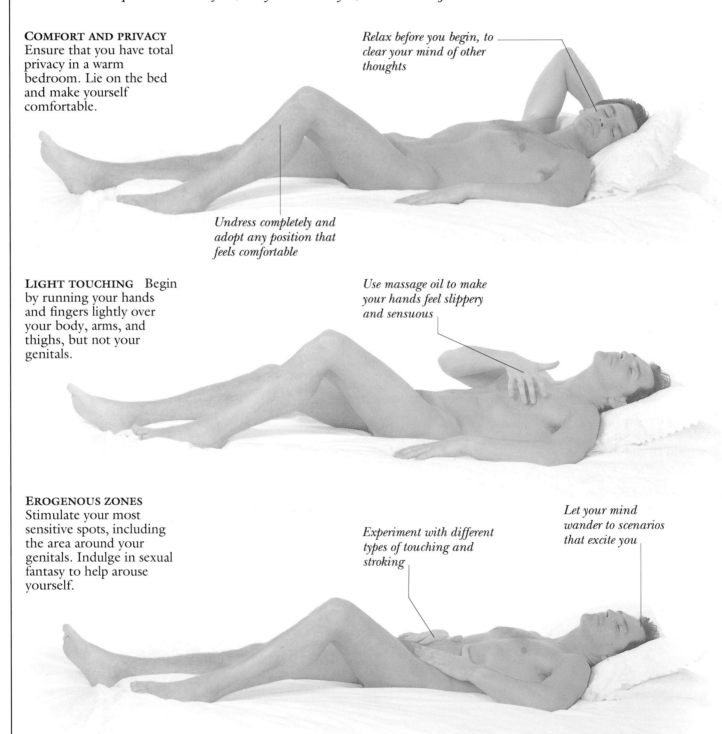

COMFORT AND PRIVACY
Ensure that you have total privacy in a warm bedroom. Lie on the bed and make yourself comfortable.

Relax before you begin, to clear your mind of other thoughts

Undress completely and adopt any position that feels comfortable

LIGHT TOUCHING Begin by running your hands and fingers lightly over your body, arms, and thighs, but not your genitals.

Use massage oil to make your hands feel slippery and sensuous

EROGENOUS ZONES
Stimulate your most sensitive spots, including the area around your genitals. Indulge in sexual fantasy to help arouse yourself.

Experiment with different types of touching and stroking

Let your mind wander to scenarios that excite you

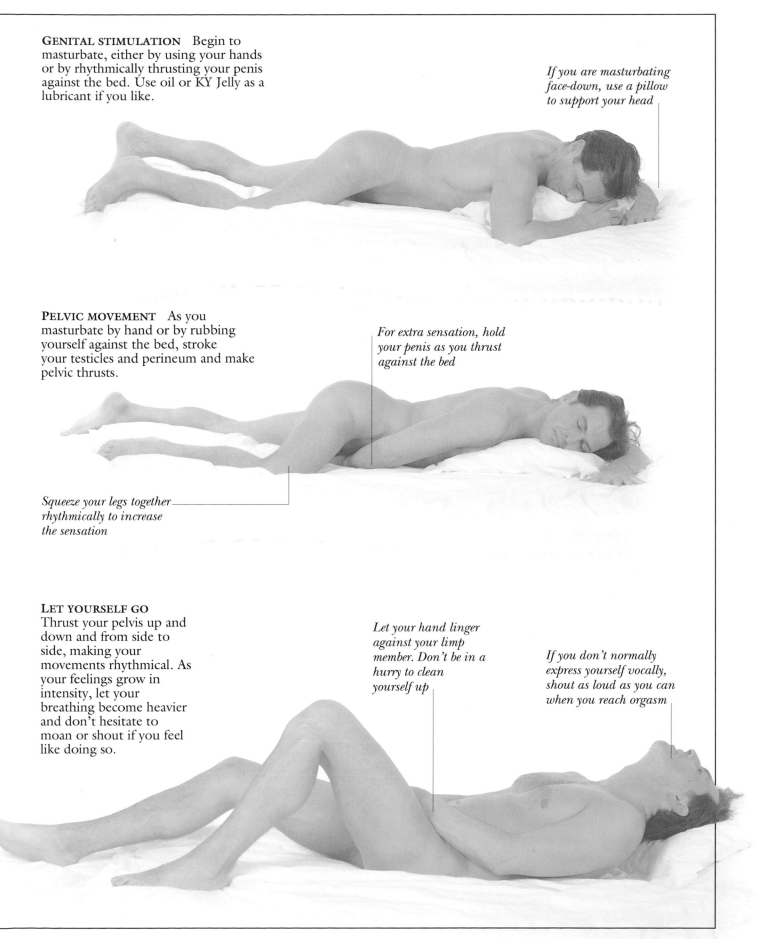

GENITAL STIMULATION   Begin to masturbate, either by using your hands or by rhythmically thrusting your penis against the bed. Use oil or KY Jelly as a lubricant if you like.

If you are masturbating face-down, use a pillow to support your head

PELVIC MOVEMENT   As you masturbate by hand or by rubbing yourself against the bed, stroke your testicles and perineum and make pelvic thrusts.

For extra sensation, hold your penis as you thrust against the bed

Squeeze your legs together rhythmically to increase the sensation

LET YOURSELF GO
Thrust your pelvis up and down and from side to side, making your movements rhythmical. As your feelings grow in intensity, let your breathing become heavier and don't hesitate to moan or shout if you feel like doing so.

Let your hand linger against your limp member. Don't be in a hurry to clean yourself up

If you don't normally express yourself vocally, shout as loud as you can when you reach orgasm

FEMALE SELF-STIMULATION

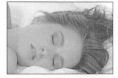 *Self-stimulation enables you to explore your body and gain detailed knowledge of your own sexual responses — knowledge that you can use as the basis of a good sexual relationship with your partner. In addition, by providing you with a solid, reliable sexual foundation upon which you can build up your self-confidence, self-stimulation can help make you feel good about yourself.*

COMFORT AND PRIVACY
Ensure that you have an hour of total privacy in a warm bedroom, and lock the door if necessary. Lie on the bed and make yourself comfortable.

LIGHT CARESSES Begin by running your hands and brushing your fingers lightly over your shoulders, arms, body, and thighs, but do not touch your genitals.

EROGENOUS ZONES
Stimulate your most sensitive spots, including your breasts and nipples but not your genitals. Indulge in sexual fantasy to help arouse yourself.

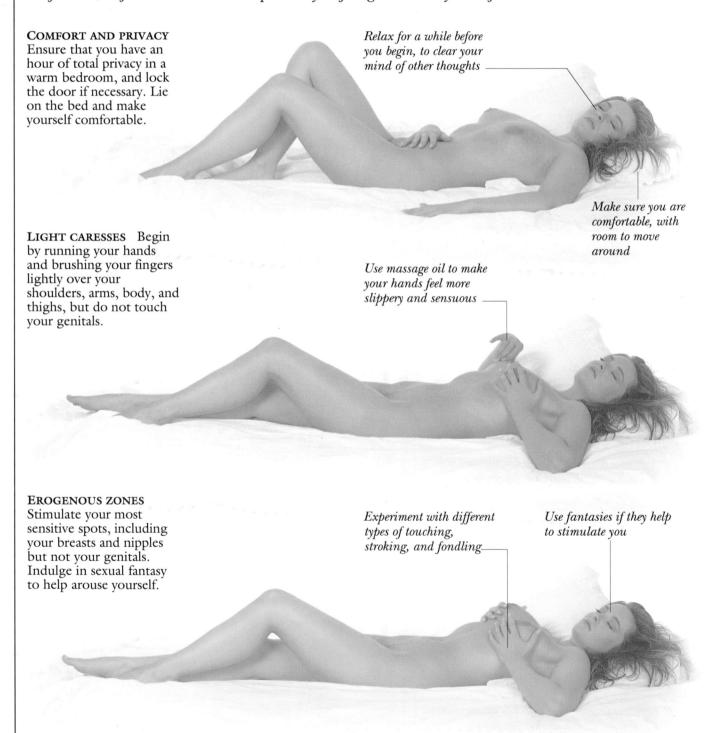

Relax for a while before you begin, to clear your mind of other thoughts

Make sure you are comfortable, with room to move around

Use massage oil to make your hands feel more slippery and sensuous

Experiment with different types of touching, stroking, and fondling

Use fantasies if they help to stimulate you

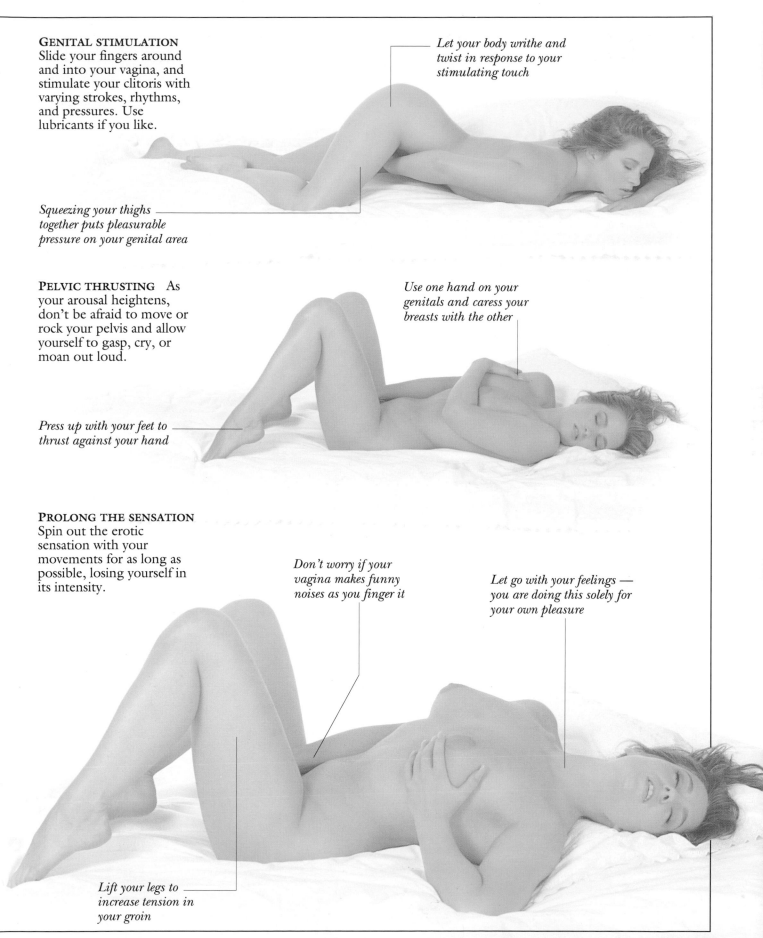

GENITAL STIMULATION
Slide your fingers around
and into your vagina, and
stimulate your clitoris with
varying strokes, rhythms,
and pressures. Use
lubricants if you like.

*Let your body writhe and
twist in response to your
stimulating touch*

*Squeezing your thighs
together puts pleasurable
pressure on your genital area*

PELVIC THRUSTING   As
your arousal heightens,
don't be afraid to move or
rock your pelvis and allow
yourself to gasp, cry, or
moan out loud.

*Use one hand on your
genitals and caress your
breasts with the other*

*Press up with your feet to
thrust against your hand*

PROLONG THE SENSATION
Spin out the erotic
sensation with your
movements for as long as
possible, losing yourself in
its intensity.

*Don't worry if your
vagina makes funny
noises as you finger it*

*Let go with your feelings —
you are doing this solely for
your own pleasure*

*Lift your legs to
increase tension in
your groin*

233

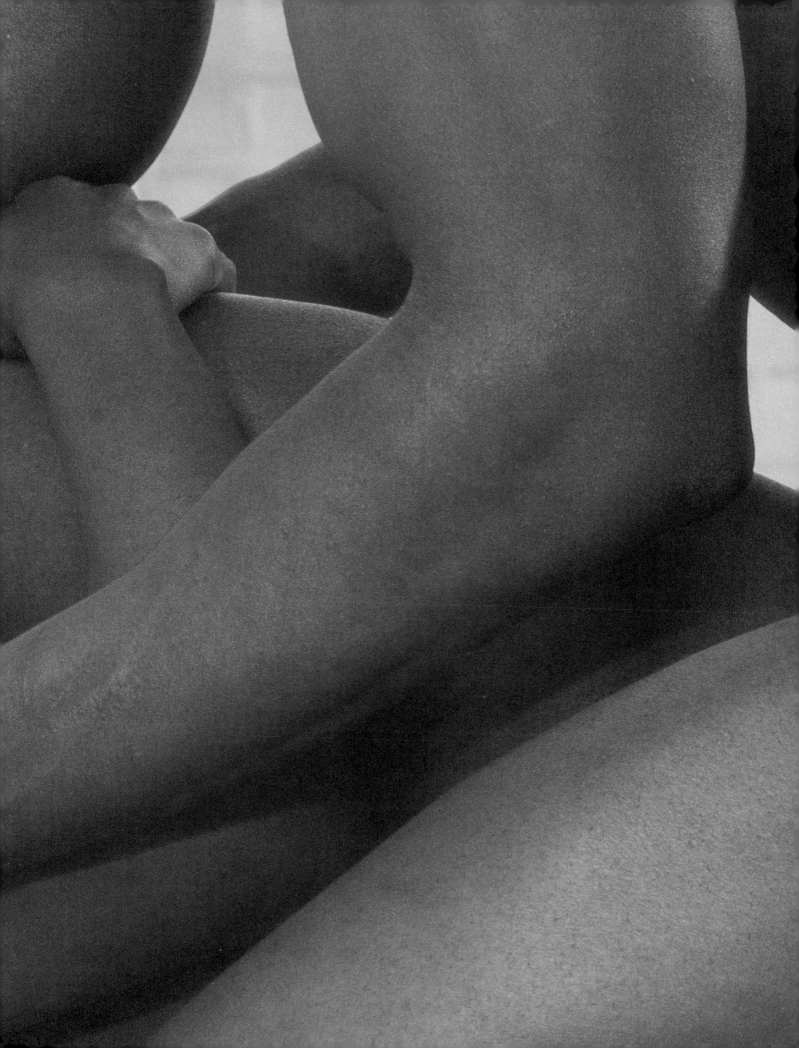

CHAPTER 22

USING SEX AIDS

"One man was so intrigued by his partner's use of a vibrator to give herself a climax that he learned to use it on her during intercourse so that she came with him inside her."

WE ARE NOT brought up to think of vibrators as natural additions to the act of sex, mainly because these objects are patently artificial. Yet vibrators, used sensitively, provide women with more stimulation than either penis or fingers and act as a catalyst to the elusive orgasm.

Vibrators are especially useful to women who suffer from what is called "automatic switch-off": because of unconscious anxiety during intercourse, their minds are distracted from sex into thinking negative thoughts that prevent climax. They may be able to become very sexually excited and reach a level — which Masters and Johnson aptly called the "plateau phase" — and from there, if they could relax mentally, they could take off into the heights of climax. But sometimes that unconscious anxiety holds them back.

In many such cases, all that the woman needs to overcome this anxiety and have an uninhibited climax is more stimulation, and the use of a vibrator will often provide her with that.

CASE STUDY *Pauline*

Pauline and her husband had an excellent relationship, and they both enjoyed sex. But Pauline rarely climaxed, and she had resorted to faking orgasms so as not to disappoint her partner, Leon, and make him feel inadequate as a lover. This strategy of faking orgasms was effective in that it encouraged Leon's self-confidence and his belief that he was a good lover, but as time went by Pauline began to feel increasingly dissatisfied at her own lack of real orgasms.

Name:	PAULINE
Age:	28
Marital status:	MARRIED
Occupation:	PHYSICAL THERAPIST

Pauline, married to Leon, a welfare officer, was sexily dressed in a low-cut blouse and was very vivacious. She and her husband had been married for three years, had no children, and were very open with each other about sexual matters.

"Leon and I make love often," she told me. "He makes me feel very sexy. But I think I've only come with him twice, and each time the orgasm has been very faint. Leon buys sex manuals and we read them together. I've taught myself to masturbate from them, and I get very turned on by some of the "dirty" stories in them. But although masturbation feels nice, I don't climax from it.

"Leon has been anxious for me to get help with this. He's very supportive. He hasn't had other lovers since we've been together, but he did once help me go to bed with a woman I liked. He took her partner out drinking so that I could go to bed with her. It was very exciting. In fact, we made love on more than one occasion. I still didn't come, though.

"Leon and I are very loving and cuddly with each other. When we're in bed together, sometimes I know I'm near orgasm. But then part of me seems to turn off at that realization. I find it hard to relax because I'm being watched by Leon. That turns me off. I'm frightened Leon is going to be so upset by my not climaxing that in the end we'll split up. I love him a great deal. I don't want that to happen.

"I have to confess that I do fake orgasm with Leon sometimes. I don't do this very often. Maybe one in four or five lovemaking sessions. I don't want him to feel he's not a success in bed. It's important for him to think of himself as a good lover. And quite frequently I feel totally satisfied by him coming. He's had such obvious pleasure from his climax and he's been so loving to me as a result of it, that I've felt a pleasure and satisfaction through him even though I myself don't technically come. But recently that hasn't been enough for me."

THERAPIST'S ASSESSMENT

What Pauline described were several common problems that get in the way of sexual enjoyment for many people. Always feeling that Leon was watching her meant that she had performance fears. When you are focusing on your performance there isn't space left in your brain to focus on heightened sensations. She needed to learn how to cut out her overawareness of Leon and focus instead on herself.

FAKING ORGASM
Faking orgasm may sometimes be expedient for the reasons Pauline outlined. But if you do it too often, it produces not only the negative effect of never allowing you to find out how to climax through intercourse, but it actually teaches your partner the wrong methods of getting you to orgasm.

Naturally, if he thinks a particular method of lovemaking works well for you, he's likely to continue using it, thereby compounding the problem. Having the courage to confess sometimes that things aren't working quite right, and asking for his patience and for different stimulation, is the road to opening up trust — and of course to orgasm. This is where vibrators can help. Sometimes, what is needed in order to get to orgasm is quite simply more stimulation. And a vibrator can provide that when a penis and fingers are flagging. But raising the subject with your partner, and persuading him to let using a vibrator become a regular part of your lovemaking, can often be a difficult move to make.

USING A VIBRATOR
I recommended that Pauline carry out the self-pleasuring program (see page 226) over a period of about four weeks, incorporating vibrator use toward the end of that time. I also suggested that she practice assertion exercises (see page 72) so that she could work up enough courage to ask Leon if they might include use of the vibrator in their lovemaking (see page 238). Use of the vibrator, plus learning to focus on some especially sexual thoughts (see page 136 on sexual fantasies), helped Pauline overcome her performance fears and reach orgasm.

My program for
INTRODUCING SEX AIDS

The answer to the question "Why use sex aids?" is "Why not?" They are fun to use, and sex should be fun as often as possible. It doesn't always have to be intense or deeply romantic or full of spiritual meaning. Sometimes it can be wonderful when it's just fooling around. And the great advantage of sex aids is that you can use them privately to assist your lighthearted experience of self-pleasuring, as well as using them on an inventive and playful partner.

Sex aids are not a recent invention: they have been around for at least the last 2,500 years. The ancient Egyptians used dildos, and a Greek vase of the fifth century B.C. shows a woman putting one enormous dildo into her mouth while a second one penetrates her vagina. The Romans made candles designed to look like huge penises, and ancient Chinese scripts tell of the custom of binding the base of the penis with silk, a method of retaining erection (an early cock ring).

The Chinese "hedgehog" was a circle of fine feathers, bound onto a silver ring that fitted over the penis. This enabled the lucky woman in question to be tickled to orgasm. Even the idea of a vibrator may have had its origin in the 1800s when female mill workers, leaning against the vibrating handles of the machinery, earned an unexpected bonus.

Sex aid prediction for the future is the sex robot. It will be programmed to overcome any sex problem — you will simply plug yourself into it and the machine will do the rest. (Remember Woody Allen and the 'Orgasmatron' in *Sleeper*?)

Stage 1 FIND OUT WHAT'S AVAILABLE

Perusal of any sex aid catalog (available from sex aid stores or by mail order through advertisements in sex magazines) will show a plethora of dildos, vibrators, cock rings, play balls, fruit-flavored massage oils and, inflatable plastic dolls, and other masturbation aids for both men and women, and usually a selection of harmless bondage items such as silken cords, blindfolds, and handcuffs. These items are relatively inexpensive and, in terms of the endless hours of enjoyment they can provide, they are generally worth the money.

DILDOS AND VIBRATORS There are any number of dildos designed in various shapes and sizes, including the double-headed dildos used by lesbian couples. The vibrator is a modern variation of the dildo and is undoubtedly the most successful sex aid ever invented.

There are vibrators that simply vibrate, and there are multispeed ones that vary in their speed of vibration from slow to supersonic. There are soft rubber ones that twist and undulate, and double ones intended for vagina and anus, with a special attachment for the clitoris, that both twist and vibrate.

There are small, slim anal vibrators with a safeguard across the top to prevent them from disappearing at an inappropriate moment. There are small cigarette-shaped vibrators designed solely for intense clitoral stimulation, and there are pink vibrating eggs which can be inserted into the vagina and switched on as you do housework or type your masterpiece.

COCK RINGS AND PLAY BALLS Cock rings are rings designed to fit closely around the base of the penis, so that the blood flow of erection is trapped inside the penis for as long as possible, should it show signs of leaking away. Play balls, or ben-wa balls, are small weighted balls for women to slip inside their vaginas, where they roll around and produce erotic sensations. The ancient Japanese were the first to use these, and Japanese women would swing in hammocks, enjoying the turn-on.

OILS, DOLLS, AND BONDAGE Fruit-flavored massage oils are specially manufactured to make oral sex tasty, and plastic inflatable dolls are designed for men and women who want to pretend they are making love to a partner when one is not available. There are versions which can be filled with hot water or, at the other end of the scale, there are rubber labia and vaginas which can claim to be "the easiest lay in the world" since they can be carried in a pocket and produced anywhere. The items of bondage equipment speak for themselves.

Despite the variety of aids now on the market, though, a vibrator is probably the best choice for a couple.

Stage 2 CHOOSING A VIBRATOR

There are two principal kinds of vibrator: those that are battery operated and those that run on electricity. The cigar-shaped battery vibrators with varying speeds of vibration are the most convenient. You don't need a great variety of heads to make their stimulation work successfully, but you do need a suitable speed of vibration.

VIBRATOR POWER Research has shown that the optimum vibration speed for facilitating a climax is 80 cycles per second. Some women need such intense stimulation, which is almost impossible to obtain by hand, and this greater frequency of vibration is best obtained on the expensive electric Japanese vibrators.

If you are using a battery-powered vibrator, invest in the long-life alkaline batteries; although these are more expensive than the standard carbon type, they are more powerful and last longer. Vibrator batteries lose power surprisingly quickly, and often, when a woman thinks she has lost the ability to climax when using her vibrator, it turns out that the batteries have run down and so the vibrator is running at well below its usual speed.

Stage 3 USING A VIBRATOR

Vibrators are a useful means of ensuring that some women climax who might otherwise never manage it. But they are also a means of enjoying wonderful clitoral sensation with-

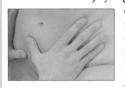

Mutual masturbation p106

out having to rely on a partner. If there is a partner in your life, it is easy to include use of a vibrator in masturbation and love play and to slip it between your bodies, focused on that strategic point, during intercourse.

What many people may not realize is that men also enjoy the sensation of vibration. There are circular vibrators, designed to slip over the penis and rest at the base, capable of bringing the man to climax too.

VIBRATORS AND LOVEMAKING Try using a warmed-up vibrator on each other's body during lovemaking. Take turns running it over each other's shoulders, neck, chest, and breasts, down the sides of the body, and around the abdomen and buttocks. Dart it in and out of the inner thighs, which for most people are sensitive erogenous zones. Explore and probe the vagina with it, and press it very gently in among the folds of the testicles and then around the base of the penis.

INTENSE SENSATIONS The areas that produce the most intense sensations when stimulated by a vibrator are the clitoris and the frenulum of the penis. The rim of the anus, for both men and women, is another good spot to stimulate, and many men get great pleasure from stimulation of the prostate, inside the anus.

VIBRATORS Vibrators are one of the most popular of all sex aids and can be used by both men and women, alone or together.

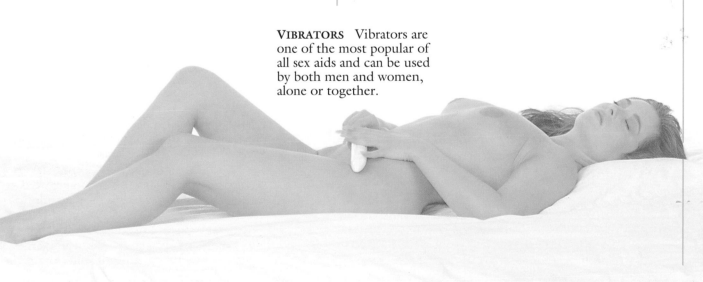

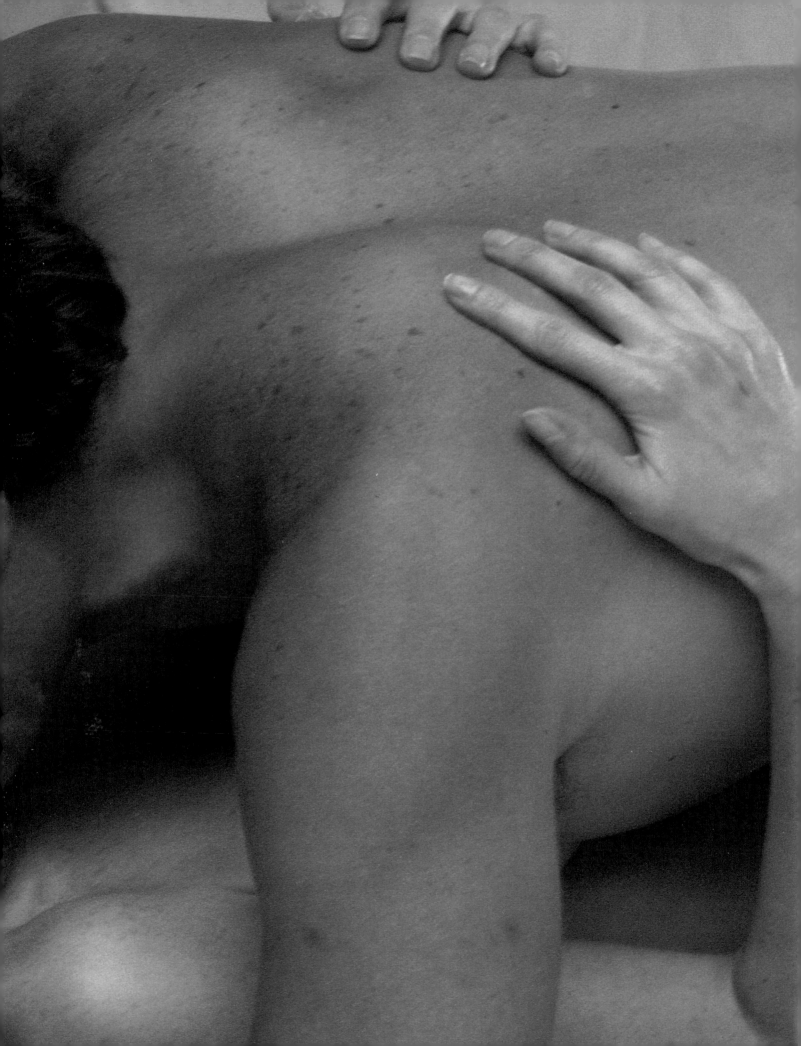

CHAPTER 23

HIS SEX ORGANS

In terms of love play and sexual intercourse, the most important single part of a man's genitals is undoubtedly his penis. However, the common belief that a man's virility and his effectiveness as a sexual partner depend on the size of his erect penis is totally misguided — what really counts is the skill and consideration with which he makes love to his partner.

MALE GENITALS The male genitals or sex organs are partly external and partly internal. The external organs are the penis and the scrotum (which contains the testicles, epididymes, and vas deferens), and the internal organs include the prostate gland and the seminal vesicles. During erection, an intricate network of vessels within the penis fills with blood, causing it to swell and stiffen. The urethra, a tube running right through the length of the penis, discharges urine from the bladder and also carries the seminal fluid during ejaculation.

GLANS The glans, the head of the penis, is rich in nerve endings which make it very sensitive to touch.

FRENULUM The highly sensitive frenulum is a small fold of skin between the glans and the shaft.

SHAFT The ridge along the underside of the penis shaft is often very sensitive to touch and stroking.

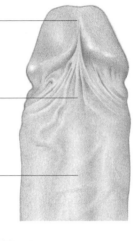

VAS DEFERENS Each vas deferens (there are two) carries sperm from the epididymis to the seminal vesicle ducts, where it is mixed with seminal fluid for ejaculation.

SEMINAL VESICLE The two seminal vesicles (one on each side of the bladder) produce most of the seminal fluid discharged during ejaculation.

Anus

PROSTATE GLAND Within the prostate gland, which is situated below the neck of the bladder, ducts from the seminal vesicles join the urethra. Manual stimulation of the gland creates intense arousal.

Bladder

Pubic bone

Penis

Urethra

Glans

Foreskin

Epididymis

TESTICLES The testicles (or testes) produce sperm and the male sex hormone testosterone. Sperm, after production, is stored in the epididymes, two long, extensively coiled ducts.

SCROTUM The scrotum has two parts. Each contains one of the testicles, suspended by a spermatic cord containing the vas deferens, blood vessels, and nerves.

HER SEX ORGANS

The external parts of a woman's genitals, and the area immediately surrounding them, are highly sensitive to physical stimulation. This sensitive region extends from the mons pubis (or mound of Venus), the padding of fatty tissue beneath the pubic hair that acts as a sort of cushion during intercourse, back to the perineum, the area between the vulva and the anus.

FEMALE GENITALS Although the female genitals are partly external, most of the organs are hidden away inside the body. The external organs (the vulva or pudendum) include the clitoris, two pairs of skin folds called the labia, and the openings of the vagina and urethra. The complex internal organs include the ovaries, fallopian tubes, uterus, cervix, and vagina. The fallopian tubes connect the ovaries to the uterus or womb, and the cervix connects the uterus to the vagina, into which the man's penis is placed during sexual intercourse.

CLITORIS The abundant nerve endings of the clitoris make it extremely sensitive to stimulation, and when stimulated it swells and becomes even more sensitive.

LABIA MAJORA The outer, larger pair of lips or skin folds that protect the openings of the vagina and urethra are the labia majora.

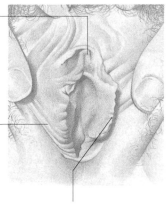

OVARIES The two ovaries each produce eggs, the female hormones estrogen and progesterone, and small amounts of testosterone.

UTERUS After an egg has been fertilized, it moves down into the uterus or womb where it eventually develops into a fetus.

LABIA MINORA The inner labia, the labia minora, secrete a substance called sebum that helps to lubricate the vagina, and they meet at the top to form the hood of the clitoris.

FALLOPIAN TUBES The fallopian tubes transport the eggs from the ovaries and the fertilization of eggs by sperm takes place within them.

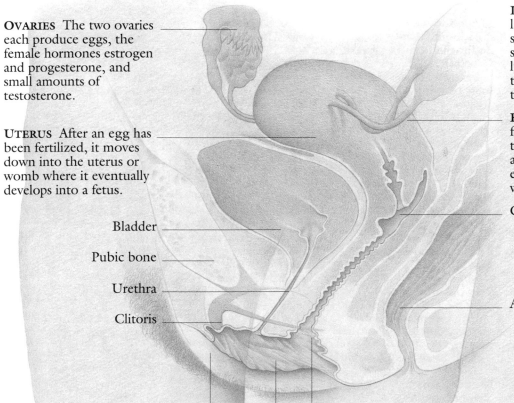

Cervix

Bladder

Pubic bone

Urethra

Clitoris

Anus

Labia majora

Vagina

Labia minora

THE ULTIMATE SEX BOOK
BENEFITED FROM:

Typesetting: Debbie Rhodes
Film outputting: DTP
Production direction: Lorraine Baird
U.S. Editor: Laaren Brown

CARROLL & BROWN LIMITED
would like to thank Bruce Garrett and
Madeline Weston for their editorial
assistance; Tim Kent and Tula Whitlow for
their photography assistance; and all the
models for the enthusiasm, cooperation and
professionalism they displayed in helping us
to produce this book.